2nd edition

101 Tips
for
Staying
Healthy with
Diabetes
(& Avoiding Complications)

University of New Mexico Diabetes Care Team

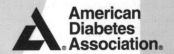

American
Diabetes
Association®

Book Acquisitions	Robert J. Anthony
Editor	Sherrye Landrum
Production Director	Carolyn R. Segree
Production Coordinator	Peggy M. Rote
Composition	Sherrye Landrum
Cover Design	Wickham & Associates, Inc.
Printer	Transcontinental Printing, Inc.

Printed in Canada

1 3 5 7 9 10 8 6 4 2

The suggestions and information contained in this publication are generally consistent with the *Clinical Practice Recommendations* and other policies of the American Diabetes Association, but they do not represent the policy or position of the Association or any of its boards or committees. Reasonable steps have been taken to ensure the accuracy of the information presented. However, the American Diabetes Association cannot ensure the safety or efficacy of any product or service described in this publication. Individuals are advised to consult a physician or other appropriate health care professional before undertaking any diet or exercise program or taking any medication referred to in this publication. Professionals must use and apply their own professional judgment, experience, and training and should not rely solely on the information contained in this publication before prescribing any diet, exercise, or medication. The American Diabetes Association—its officers, directors, employees, volunteers, and members—assumes no responsibility or liability for personal or other injury, loss, or damage that may result from the suggestions or information in this publication.

ADA titles may be purchased for business or promotional use or for special sales. For information, please write to Lee M. Romano, Special Sales & Promotions, at the address below.

American Diabetes Association
1660 Duke Street
Alexandria, Virginia 22314

Library of Congress Cataloging-in-Publication Data

101 tips for staying healthy with diabetes (& avoiding
complications) : a project of the American Diabetes Association /
written and produced by The University of New Mexico Diabetes Care
Team ; David S. Schade, editor in chief ... [et al.]. -- 2nd ed.
    p. cm.
  ISBN 1-58040-007-8 (pbk.)
  1. Diabetes Popular works. 2. Diabetes Miscellanea. 3.
Diabetes--Complications--Prevention Miscellanea. I. Schade, David
S., 1942- II. University of New Mexico. Diabetes Care Team. III.
American Diabetes Association. IV. Title: One hundred tips for
staying healthy with diabetes (& avoiding complications) V. Title:
One hundred one tips for staying healthy with diabetes (& avoiding
complications)
RC660.4 .A16 1999
616.4'62--dc21   99--22930
                                                         CIP

101 TIPS FOR STAYING HEALTHY WITH DIABETES (& AVOIDING COMPLICATIONS)

▼

TABLE OF CONTENTS

ACKNOWLEDGMENTS

▼

The University of New Mexico Diabetes Care Team thanks Carolyn King, MEd, of the University of New Mexico for her editorial expertise and hard work on the manuscripts. We also acknowledge the editorial assistance of Sherrye Landrum of the American Diabetes Association and the graphic expertise of Wickham & Associates for the cover design of this series.

Thanks to Greg Edmondson and Aime Ballard-Wood for copyediting the two editions of this book and to Francine Kaufman, MD; Eleanor Lordon, RN, MS, CNS, CDE; Lea Ann Holzmeister, RN, CDE; and David Kelley, MD, for reviewing the manuscripts. A special thanks to Jim Stein of Insight Graphics for desktopping the first edition of this book. Carolyn Segree coordinated printing of the first edition, and Peggy Rote handled the printing of the second edition.

Introduction

▼

We were very pleased that our first book, *101 Tips for Improving Your Blood Sugar*, was so well received by people with diabetes. This first book was the result of suggestions made to us by our patients who had successfully found ways to reduce their blood sugars to appropriate target ranges. We then passed these suggestions on to you, our readers. The current book, *101 Tips for Staying Healthy with Diabetes (& Avoiding Complications),* brings more of our patients' tips to you.

We have revised this book to be certain that all tips are current. Diabetes care changes rapidly and new information becomes available daily. We have replaced out-of-date tips and added an extra ten tips to the book to provide you with new information.

As health providers, we are convinced that the patient has to make the important decisions concerning diabetes and health. To do this successfully, you must understand both the reasons for the health goals and ways to accomplish them. Diabetes treatment is undergoing rapid changes, and our books are formatted to help you find and remember the information you need more easily. Thanks to many dedicated individuals and organizations, additional options for treatment will continue to become available in the future. We are grateful to the American Diabetes Association for publishing our books and making them available to its members at reduced cost. All proceeds from our books go to furthering diabetes care and research. With your help, we believe that diabetes will be a "curable" disease within the next 10 years. Thank you.

—The University of New Mexico Diabetes Care Team

Chapter 1
GENERAL INFORMATION

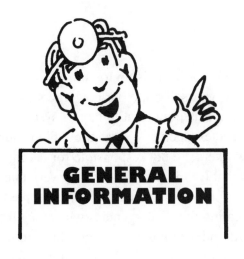

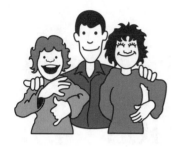

Should I tell my boss and coworkers that I have diabetes?

▼
TIP:

Whether or not to tell anyone is up to you. You do have a responsibility to yourself and your coworkers to keep the work environment safe. It is important to have a system in place for managing emergencies, such as a severe low blood sugar or a sick day. Your coworkers are not responsible for taking care of you, but you will probably find that they will be very understanding and want to help you stay healthy. Most people feel more comfortable dealing with emergencies when they have some preparation and understanding. You don't have to make diabetes the daily topic of conversation, and you may feel uncomfortable letting people at work become the "control patrol." This is a personal choice that requires consideration on your part, but you will find that your life is easier if you allow others to support you in managing your diabetes and staying healthy.

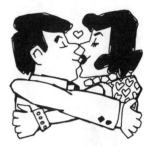

*C*an I catch diabetes from someone
 else?

▼
TIP:

No, you cannot. Diabetes is not like a cold or the flu. There are many causes of diabetes, but neither type 1 nor type 2 has ever been shown to be infectious or contagious (catchable). You cannot catch diabetes from another person, even by kissing them. Most diabetes develops from an inherited tendency to get it. If you have inherited this gene, you may develop type 1 diabetes when you are exposed to something in the environment. This unknown factor triggers the onset of diabetes. You may develop type 2 diabetes if (in addition to inheriting the gene) you gain weight and don't exercise regularly. There are also less common causes of diabetes, such as prolonged, excessive drinking of alcohol or having too much iron in your blood. Thus, there are many causes of diabetes, but catching it from another person is not one of them.

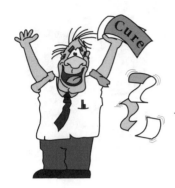

*H*ow close are we to a cure for diabetes?

▼
TIP:

It depends on what you mean by "cure." Diabetes is not really one disease. It probably has many causes and, therefore, many cures. Much progress has been made in the last few years toward prevention of diabetes and treatment of the disease once it occurs. These advances are important until cures are available. The ultimate cure for diabetes would probably be a replacement for the cells of the pancreas that make insulin. This could be done by inserting a remote-controlled insulin pump that is automatically regulated by a glucose sensor. The implantable pump has already been developed and tested in more than 400 people worldwide. Glucose sensors are under development and should be available soon.

Another approach is to transplant insulin-producing cells into the person with diabetes. This approach has already been done successfully in animals with diabetes. It has been more difficult in humans, because our body sees these cells as foreign material and tends to kill them off. Many researchers are trying to overcome these problems. What we can say is that we expect a cure for some types of diabetes within the next 10 years.

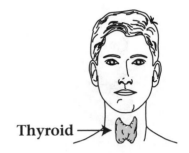

Thyroid ——▶

*D*oes diabetes put me at risk for developing thyroid problems?

▼
TIP:

Perhaps. The thyroid gland in your neck secretes thyroid hormone. Low levels of thyroid hormone (thyroid failure) are common in individuals with type 1 diabetes. Thyroid hormone gives you energy and helps maintain other organ systems in your body. We recommend that you get a blood test for thyroid hormone once a year, particularly if you feel more tired than usual or have other symptoms such as constipation, dry skin, and feeling cold most of the time. Treatment is easy and inexpensive. This is important, because when low thyroid hormone goes untreated, it can lead to many medical problems. Do not hesitate to ask your doctor periodically to check your blood thyroid hormone level. Remember that other medical problems can occur in people with diabetes that are not directly related to high blood sugar levels.

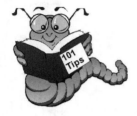

How can I make the most of my visit with my health care team?

▼
TIP:

First, plan ahead. Write down on paper all the questions that you want to ask the team. It is too easy to forget your questions if you don't write them down. Also bring along a pencil or pen to write down the answers. If you're prepared, the visit is more likely to meet your needs. Second, show up for your appointment on time. If you are late, your health care team may not be able to spend enough time with you to solve your problems. (For waiting room reading, you could bring this book or our first book, *101 Tips for Improving Your Blood Sugar*, and review the tips that apply to you.) Third, always bring in all your current medications so that the health care team can check them. This will ensure that you don't run out of medication and that the pharmacy gives you the medication that your doctor prescribes. Fourth, be sure to bring in records of your recent blood sugars, weight, blood pressure, and exercise schedule. These records help you and the team see your progress in meeting your goals. If you don't have a logbook, bring your blood glucose meter.

*H*ow often should I plan on seeing
*my doctor to be as healthy as I
can be?*

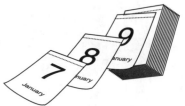

▼
TIP:

The frequency of medical visits required for your diabetes will vary according to how long you've had diabetes, your ability to adjust your treatment regimen effectively to maintain good blood sugar control, and whether you have diabetic complications or other medical problems that may interfere with your diabetes management.

At a minimum, all diabetic patients should plan on seeing a doctor twice a year. Recharging your motivation to achieve good blood sugar control is an important part of every visit. You should have an HbA_{1c} test done then, or if you are on insulin, you should have the test done quarterly to see how your blood glucose control is doing.

In addition, every patient with diabetes should have someone they can contact on short notice to discuss problems as they arise, such as unexplained high blood sugars or sudden illness. This person need not be a physician but may be a certified diabetes educator (CDE), registered dietitian (RD), nurse practitioner, or nurse case manager.

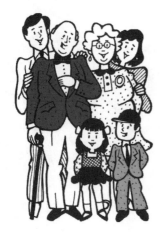

*S*hould members of my family
read this book?

▼
TIP:

Yes! There are several good reasons for each member of your family to read this book. First, there are many tips that apply equally well to people without diabetes. Anyone who wants to stay in good health will benefit from these tips. Second, your family members can support you better when they understand what is needed. For example, a change to eating healthier meals is easier if all family members make the same commitment. There are outdated ideas of what is good for a person with diabetes. Keeping up-to-date makes it easier to plan family outings, picnics, and parties with you in mind. Each family member should be able to recognize the signs and symptoms of low blood sugar. Third, family members of people with diabetes have a higher risk of developing diabetes themselves. By changing to a healthier lifestyle, you and your family members, we believe, will prevent or significantly delay the onset of diabetes.

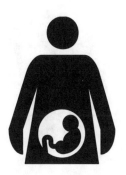

*D*oes getting diabetes when I am *pregnant mean that I am more likely to get permanent diabetes later?*

▼
TIP:

Yes. The fact that you get high blood sugars during pregnancy indicates that your pancreas cannot make enough extra insulin to cover the increased needs caused by pregnancy. This suggests that you might develop diabetes even if you never get pregnant again. Approximately 5% of women like you will develop diabetes each year if they don't make efforts to improve their lifestyles. Women gain weight during pregnancy but do not always lose all of it after delivery. With several pregnancies, a woman may gain quite a bit of weight. Therefore, if you develop high blood sugars during pregnancy, it is most important that you lose all of the weight you gained during your pregnancy. Eat healthy meals and exercise daily. This is the best approach you can take to prevent permanent diabetes from occurring.

If you decide to breastfeed, do not begin a weight-loss program without medical advice. To breastfeed you need the same amount of calories that you needed during the last 3 months of your pregnancy. When you stop breastfeeding, then you can focus on losing any extra weight that you still have.

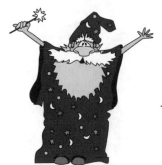

*I*s diabetes a new disease?

▼
TIP:

No. Diabetes was known more than 2,000 years ago when Aretaeus of Cappadocia, the Greek physician, named it. However, very little progress was made in understanding or treating the disease until 1869, when Paul Langerhans described small islands (islets) in the pancreas. However, he did not know their function. Things progressed more rapidly when Oskar Minkowski realized that removing the pancreas from a dog caused the dog to urinate frequently. He also found sugar in the dog's urine. In 1909, the Belgian scientist Jean de Meyer used the term "insulin" for a hypothetical substance in the pancreas that controlled blood sugar even though insulin had not yet been discovered. Finally in 1921, after a series of experiments, J.J.R. Macleod, Charles Best, Frederick Banting, and James Collip succeeded in purifying insulin and successfully treating a diabetic patient with it. This discovery saved many people from dying in a coma caused by high blood sugars. Diabetes has been around a long time, but we still need new and better therapies.

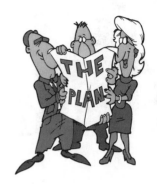

*W*hat is my "health care team" and how can I find these health providers?

▼
TIP:

In addition to your doctor, you need someone trained to help you with the day-to-day challenges of living with diabetes. Diabetes educator nurses and dietitians, plus your doctor, are the core members of your health care team. A certified diabetes educator (CDE) is a health professional (registered nurse [RN], registered dietitian [RD], pharmacist, physician, etc.) who has been trained and "certified" as an expert in diabetes education and management. If you cannot find a CDE, you may find a nurse or an RD interested in diabetes and willing to help you. Ask your doctor if he or she knows someone with diabetes experience. You can locate a CDE in your area by calling the American Association of Diabetes Educators (AADE) Diabetes Educator Access Line at (800) 832-6874. They will ask for your zip code and help you find a CDE near you. You may also want to look for a diabetes-education program that offers individual or group classes. The American Diabetes Association has a list of "recognized" diabetes programs and there may be one in your area. Call (800) DIABETES for this information. If there isn't a recognized diabetes center near you, call your local hospital and ask about a diabetes education program or diabetes educators on staff.

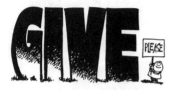

What can I do to help cure diabetes?

▼
TIP:

You can do a lot! Most people don't realize how important their effort can be in helping to cure diabetes. The main reason that so much progress has been made in the last 50 years is the work of individuals like you supporting organizations searching for the cures for diabetes. One of these organizations is the American Diabetes Association (ADA).

At the local level, you can encourage friends and neighbors to support fundraising efforts by your local ADA offices, such as walking events. Donations support new research in diabetes and are deductible from your income tax. Joining will connect you to up-to-date information on better diabetes management and keep you informed of important legislation concerning diabetes in the U.S. Congress. Your letters to your local and state representatives (congressmen and senators) can definitely help make state and national monies available for diabetes research and treatment. Your local ADA office ([888] DIABETES) can provide you with their names and addresses. Remember, you really can make a difference.

*I*s diabetes a dangerous disease?

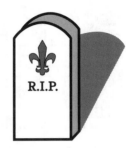

▼
TIP:

Yes, it is. There are statistics to prove that diabetes causes much suffering and loss of time from work. For example, it is the leading cause of kidney failure in this country. In addition, 15,000 to 30,000 people each year lose their eyesight because of diabetes. This year 160,000 individuals will die from diabetes-related causes in the United States. In fact, according to experts, during the last 20 years, diabetes has caused more deaths than all of the wars throughout the world in the last century. Unfortunately, the situation is getting worse, not better, because of the increasing number of people developing diabetes. We all need to do our best to prevent and to treat this disease in the U.S. and throughout the world.

The results of the Diabetes Control and Complications Trial (DCCT) and the United Kingdom Prospective Diabetes Study (UKPDS) show that you can live a healthier life with diabetes by keeping blood glucose levels near normal. Modern advances in self-testing and treatment make this possible.

		D	E	M	E	T	R	I	U	S
		I								
S	U	G	A	R		U				
		B		R		R				
	M	E	L	L	I	T	U	S		
		T		N		W				
W	A	T	E	R		E				
		S		E		L				
						L				

*W*hat does the name diabetes
mellitus mean?

▼
TIP:

T he names diabetes and mellitus come from two different
places. The first name, diabetes, is usually attributed to the
Greek physician Aretaeus, who lived in 200 B.C. He used the
term diabetes, meaning siphon or to flow through, for a disease
in which the water that a person drinks runs rapidly through his
or her body. His patients sucked up water at one end and emp-
tied it at the other. It was not until the end of the 18th century
that the term mellitus was added to diabetes. An Englishman,
John Rollo, and a German, Johann Peter Frank, first used the
term mellitus (which means sweet as honey) in the medical liter-
ature to describe the sweet taste of the urine. So, to answer your
question, the name diabetes mellitus means a medical condition
in which the patient drinks too much water and urinates frequently. The urine is sweet because it contains sugar.

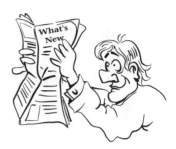

*H*ow can I know whether a new
diabetes product is right for me?

▼
TIP:

This is one time when being a skeptic is a good idea. Many
times, news releases make a product sound like it will work
for everyone, but in fact it may only be useful for specific conditions. In the United States, we have many regulations to protect
us from unproven (and possibly dangerous) new treatments. The
Food and Drug Administration (FDA) has strict guidelines
regarding the research and testing that must be done on a new
drug or therapy before it can be sold to the public. Many times
you will read reports about a new product or drug, but it is still
in the early phases of testing. Testing takes several years. If
safety problems or side effects are found during the testing, the
product will not be marketed. Your health care team may have
information on new products, so you should check with them
when something new is available. They will help you make a
decision as to whether the new product is right for you.

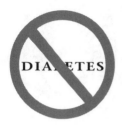 *Can diabetes be prevented?*

▼
TIP:

Many scientists believe that the answer is "yes." Because the causes of type 1 and type 2 diabetes are different, approaches to preventing each form of diabetes are different.

Type 1 diabetes is thought to be caused by an allergic-like reaction, probably to insulin, the pancreas, or some substance in the pancreas. If this is true, then it is possible that diabetes could be prevented by giving the susceptible person small injections of insulin, much like allergy shots may prevent hay fever. This approach has been successful in animals who were bred to get diabetes. The National Institutes of Health (NIH) is currently conducting a nationwide study to test this promising possibility.

Type 2 diabetes does not seem to be caused by an allergic reaction. The cause is probably related to an inherited defect that reduces a person's sensitivity to insulin. New medications used early may prevent type 2 diabetes. Also, lifestyle changes (exercise and weight loss) may reverse this defect and prevent it. The U.S. government is testing this promising approach in another nationwide study. Within the next 5 to 10 years, we should know the answer to your question.

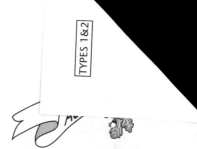

*I*s there a time of year when people
are more likely to get diabetes?

▼
TIP:

Yes and no. Many studies have been done to determine when people get diabetes.

Type 1 diabetes (previously called "insulin-dependent diabetes") usually occurs in individuals less than 30 years of age. It is more common to develop type 1 diabetes in the fall of the year, which happens to be the season in which many viral infections occur (for example, chicken pox, flu, and measles). The higher rate of type 1 diabetes during the fall months has been used to suggest that type 1 diabetes may be started by a virus that causes an infection. Whether this is true or not has not been found.

Type 2 diabetes (previously called "non-insulin-dependent diabetes") usually occurs in overweight people over the age of 30 years. There does not seem to be a seasonal increase in the development of type 2 diabetes. This difference in the time of year that diabetes develops is one of the many ways the two types of diabetes are not alike.

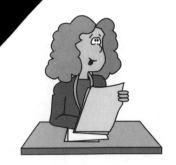

Why do I have a preexisting condition rider attached to my health insurance policy that excludes any coverage for my diabetes for 1 year?

▼

TIP:

Insurance companies separate people into groups depending on their "risk" (the chance that they will cost money to the insurance company). Because diabetes is expensive to manage and because diabetes is associated with other serious diseases, insurance companies feel that they should either charge you more or not cover you for the first year. In this first year with preexisting conditions excluded, you must try to find a way to protect yourself from excessive health care expenses. Before you change jobs, be sure to consider the complete health benefit package of both jobs. Consider the impact your new job may have on your present health benefits package. You may be able to retain insurance coverage from your previous position by selecting your COBRA benefit, which is required by law to allow you to continue your insurance for 18 months. You should also check with your state insurance commission to find out if your state has an insurance program for people who are uninsurable because they have a chronic disease. If you are unable to afford insurance or health care costs, many county- or state-supported hospitals have funds that are available to help with medical costs.

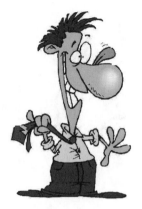

*W*ill Viagra help me if my impotence is *due to diabetes?*

▼
TIP:

Maybe. As you are aware, Viagra is the only FDA-approved oral medication for impotence (erectile dysfunction) in the United States. This medication has proved safe, and 65–85% of men using it report an improvement in erections. Please note that Viagra does not increase the desire for sex, only the ability to maintain an erection. In one study that focused exclusively on men whose impotence was attributed to diabetes, the men kept diaries throughout the study. These diaries demonstrated that approximately 50% of attempts at sexual intercourse were successful for men taking Viagra but only about 10% were successful for those taking a placebo. Side effects of Viagra include headaches, facial flushing, and indigestion, but there has been no evidence of an effect on a person's glucose control. No one should take Viagra if he is also taking a nitroglycerin or nitrate in any form, because dangerous low blood pressure may result. If you have heart disease or are taking other medications, talk with your health provider about whether this product is safe for you to use.

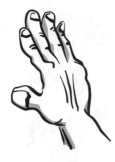

*W*hy are my fingernails thick and pulling
away from the nail bed?

▼
TIP:

You may have a fungal infection of your fingernails. Fungal infections of the skin, such as "athlete's foot," are more common in people with diabetes. These fungal infections can occasionally involve unusual areas of the body, such as your nails, scalp, or groin. A fungal infection of your fingernails is not a serious threat to your overall health, but it may make your nails brittle and unsightly. You can also spread the infection to other areas of your body, such as your scalp, by scratching with infected nails.

You should see your health care team or a dermatologist (skin specialist) to have your infection treated. They can take a sample from under your nails and examine it under the microscope to confirm the diagnosis. Nail infections are difficult to cure, and you will probably require treatment with an oral drug for several months. Because these drugs may damage your liver or bone marrow, you may need to have blood tests every few weeks to monitor your blood cell counts and your liver function. After all of this effort, you may be rewarded with the return of healthy nails.

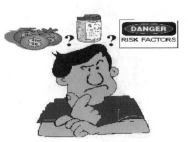

*W*hich type 2 medication should I use?

▼
TIP:

You and your health care provider must discuss this. There are several different classes of medicine for the treament of diabetes, and the one you should use depends on dosing requirements, side effects, low blood sugar risk, cost, and (most importantly) whether or not it enables you to meet your target blood glucose goals. If you are unable to meet your target goals with only one agent, your health provider may place you on two or more drugs to try to control your diabetes.

Generic Name	Dosing and Side Effects	Hypo-glycemia Risk	Cost
Glipizide (Glucotrol), Glyburide (Micronase, Diabeta) Glimepiride (Amaryl)	1–2 times a day	Medium	Low
Metformin (Glucophage)	1–2 times a day. Causes gas, bloating, or diarrhea in 20–30% of cases	Low	Medium
Repaglinide (Prandin)	3 times a day	Medium	Medium
Troglitazone (Rezulin)	1 time a day. Causes rare liver problems and requires monthly blood testing	Low	High
Acarbose (Precose)	3 times a day. Causes gas bloating, and diarrhea in up to 50% of cases	Low	Medium
Insulin injections	1–3 times a day	High	Low

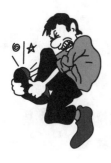

Should I be concerned about a small red blister on my foot from walking in new shoes?

▼
TIP:

Yes! You may look at a small blister and think that it is nothing serious, but it can be. If it breaks, this blister in the skin can allow germs into your foot. These germs can cause an infection not only in your foot, but also in the bone. Infections in the bone are very difficult to treat and often are the cause of amputations. What you should do right now is to wash your feet carefully in gentle soap and water and dry them thoroughly. Then put a small amount of antibiotic ointment on a dressing and cover the wound. Next, call your health care team and let them know that you have a sore on your foot. Your health care team will want to see your foot to decide whether you need to get started on an antibiotic medication. Finally, quit wearing the shoes that caused the blister. Purchasing a comfortable pair of shoes is one of the best investments you can make. The shoes you wear must fit your feet. Careful attention can prevent future problems.

*A*m I more likely to develop skin infections
*A*because I have diabetes?

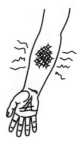

▼
TIP:

Y ou may be. People with diabetes who are overweight or
who have high blood sugars most of the time are more
likely to develop skin infections than are thin people with normal blood sugars. High blood sugars can interfere with your
body's natural defense systems. Once they start, some of these
infections can spread rapidly, causing fever, chills, and tiredness. It is very important that you examine your skin each day
and promptly take care of any sores, redness, or skin break-
downs that may be new. Yeast infections usually occur in
warm, moist areas of the body, particularly in the genital
region, under breasts, and between folds of skin. Infections of
the face, foot, and ear canal may be particularly serious and
should be checked by your health care team. Many different
types of treatment are available for these skin problems, and
you should ask for advice before applying drugstore skin
creams. Good skin care is essential for good health.

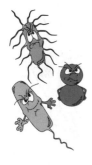

*C*an my diabetes cause diarrhea?

▼
TIP:

Yes. Frequent diarrhea occurs in 5–20% of people with long-standing diabetes. The possible causes include fewer digestive enzymes being released from the pancreas, overuse of magnesium-containing antacids, or too many bacteria in the upper part of the intestine (where they should not normally be). Often, however, the cause is unknown. Damage to the nerves that control movement in the bowel is thought to be a basic cause. Have an evaluation by your health care team. For example, if you don't have enough digestive enzymes, a pill taken with meals may cure the problem. If the cause of your diarrhea remains unknown, there are still treatments that may increase the hardness of your stools and decrease the number of daily bowel movements. Some of these treatments include simple over-the-counter remedies like psyllium (Metamucil) or a kaolin and pectin mixture (Kaopectate). Other people respond to prescription drugs, such as cholesterol-binding resins (cholestyramine), antibiotics (tetracycline or erythromycin), or drugs designed to decrease movement in the bowel (loperamide [Lomotil]). Whatever the cause of your diarrhea, you deserve a careful medical review of this problem, because chances are good that some of your symptoms can be relieved.

*C*ould I lose my job driving a
truck if I start insulin?

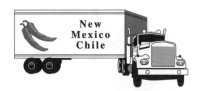

▼
TIP:

If you can prove that your diabetes is in good control with
detailed blood glucose records and glycated hemoglobin
(HbA$_{1c}$) test results, you may be able to continue in the job in
your state. Individual state governments have rules for jobs
driving automobiles, trucks, or commercial vehicles within that
state. Most jobs are reviewed on a case-by-case basis.

However, the U.S. Department of Transportation Federal
Highway Administration governs driving commercial vehicles
between states. Their policy is that "a person is physically
qualified to drive a motor vehicle if he or she has no
established medical history or clinical diagnosis of diabetes
mellitus currently requiring insulin for control." This would
prevent you from driving a truck across state lines if you are
taking insulin. You should contact your state Department of
Transportation to see what the policy is for various
occupations that rely on driving ability within that state.

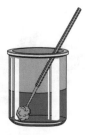

Should I test my urine for glucose and ketones?

▼
TIP:

Sometimes. Urine testing is not an accurate way to measure blood sugar. It is the way to check for ketones when you cannot eat or are ill. A buildup of ketones tells you that you are developing ketoacidosis. Ketones are breakdown products of fat that produce acid in the body. Too much acid can result in your being hospitalized. Therefore, when you are sick with a cold or the flu, you should test your urine for ketones and call your health care team if you detect any. You can buy urine ketone testing strips at the drugstore.

The information about blood glucose that you get from urine testing for sugar is not precise enough to make decisions for treatment. Your kidney does not spill sugar into your urine until your blood sugar is higher than 200 mg/dl. The ADA does not recommend that you use urine sugar testing (especially if you're taking insulin) if you can perform finger-stick blood glucose testing.

*W*here can I find information about
diabetes on the Internet?

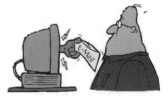

▼
TIP:

There are numerous places to find information about diabetes. The first to consider is the ADA Web site
(www.diabetes.org). This site gives you information to help
you understand the causes and treatment of diabetes. In addition, the Centers for Disease Control and Prevention (CDC)
home page (www.CDC.gov) offers extensive information
about chronic diseases, including diabetes. You can find
statistics on the incidence and prevalence of diabetes and its
complications and a patient guide called *Take Charge of Your
Diabetes*. This manual can be downloaded free of charge. The
CDC site also has a traveler's health information page, which
includes material for international travelers, geographical
health recommendations, and vaccine information. Diabetes
information can also be found at the NIH Web site
(www.nih.gov), including the home page for the National
Institute of Diabetes and Digestive and Kidney Diseases
(NIDDK) (www.niddk.nih.gov). This Web site offers a nice
glossary and definition of many diabetes-related terms. This
site is also linked to *Diabetes in America,* 2nd Edition, which
contains extensive public information on diabetes in the United
States. These sites should answer most of your diabetes questions.

Chapter 2
GLUCOSE CONTROL

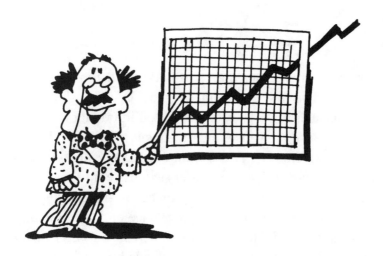

*W*hy can't I get my 8-year-old daughter to help take care of her diabetes?

▼
TIP:

B ecause it is difficult and frustrating for her to do it. Young children usually are unable to assume full responsibility for their diabetes care until they reach the teenage years. In fact, an 8-year-old child cannot understand something as complicated as a chronic disease, and she may actually blame herself for the fact that she has diabetes. She may be more timid than other children her age and worry more than usual when you are apart from her ("separation anxiety").

She has new and challenging tasks every day, like going to school and making new friends, so she may not be interested in caring for her diabetes. She needs to feel secure in her daily activities and let you care for her diabetes for now. It may help her self-confidence if she succeeds at doing some of the basic tasks such as blood glucose checks and keeping her log book. Discuss with your health care team how flexible her schedule can be and the appropriate goals for her diabetes control. You may find that you can loosen up on her control somewhat in the interest of safety and convenience. Remember that the day is coming when your daughter will be able to care for her diabetes herself, and she'll only need your help occasionally. Just don't rush her.

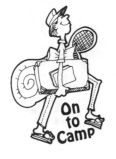

On to Camp

How can I help my 13-year-old son cope with his diabetes?

▼
TIP:

This is a hectic period in his life with rapid changes inside and out, and diabetes care may be low on his priority list. The onset of puberty can complicate diabetes care. He may have a dramatic increase in insulin requirements over a short period of time. Turn over the responsibility for diabetes care to your son gradually as he is ready to accept it. You will both need to be flexible to adjust to all the demands on him.

It is possible that your son may be more open to learning from his peers than from you during the coming years. Help him get together with other teenagers who have diabetes so that he can see the various ways they cope with diabetes. Diabetes summer camp provides an excellent opportunity for this. Your son will see both healthy and unhealthy behaviors at camp, but he'll be encouraged to manage his own diabetes with experience and knowledge. Most states have a diabetes summer camp with a full medical staff. The friendships that develop at camp are often strong and can last a lifetime. Contact the ADA at (888) DIABETES (342-2383) for more information about a camp in your area.

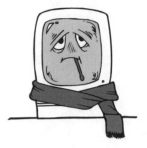

*W*hat can I take for a cold, since it seems that all the cold medicines at the drugstore are labeled "not for people with diabetes"?

▼
TIP:

Probably the best thing to do about a cold is to take aceta-minophen (Tylenol) for the aches, pains, or fever; get plenty of rest; and drink lots of fluids. Be sure to check your blood sugar often and be ready to respond to a rise in your blood sugar. You and your health care team need to set up a sick-day plan. Then you'll know better what to eat or drink, when to test your blood glucose and ketones, and when to call them for help.

Drugs that help reduce the symptoms of a cold are cough medicines, antihistamines (which blocks allergic reactions), and decongestants (which reduce swelling in the nose). The cough medicines and antihistamines may make you very sleepy. Chemicals in decongestants work in your swollen sinus tissues by making the blood vessels narrower and thus reducing blood flow. This may help your runny nose, but if you have heart disease or very poor circulation, they can cause serious problems. If you have diabetes, the label warns you to talk to your doctor before taking this medicine.

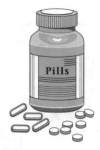

Will the medication I am taking for depression affect my blood sugar?

▼
TIP:

Probably not. Depression is more common in patients with chronic diseases like diabetes—up to 40% of people with diabetes may have depression at some point in their lives. Medications for depression have no major direct impact on how your oral diabetes medication or insulin works to control your blood sugar.

On the other hand, keeping diabetes management at the top of your list of things to deal with can seem impossible if you are depressed. A vicious cycle can develop in which high blood sugars make you feel sleepy and as though you don't have enough energy to get out and exercise. The exercise would help bring the blood glucose down and make you feel better physically and mentally. Dealing with depression can break the cycle and put you back on track, eating right and exercising, to help you feel better all the time. While there are many ways of dealing with depression, sometimes several months of treatment with medication can allow you to get back to being yourself faster.

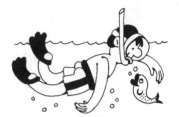

I have arthritis in my hips; can you recommend exercises other than walking?

▼
TIP:

Many people with arthritic pain in their hips or knees cannot take the 30- to 60-minute walk each day that is recommended to improve blood sugar control. You can do armchair aerobics and stretches while sitting. Water aerobics in a swimming pool is another activity that does not put stress on your joints. If you can do them, gentle "standing" exercises such as tai chi or chi kung can give you a no-impact workout. All exercise routines should include a 10-minute warm-up period, 10–30 minutes of exercise, and a 10-minute cool-down period. The exercise must be intense enough to get your heart rate up, but not so intense that you can't speak. You may break out in a light sweat (if you're not in a pool).

Weight loss or maintaining a weight loss is not the only benefit of exercising. Exercise also increases insulin sensitivity, improves blood flow to the heart and muscles, and helps improve blood sugar control. As with all exercise programs, you should consult your health care team for recommendations about the activity that is right for you. Don't let your arthritis prevent you from exercising.

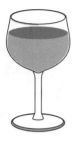

*I*s it acceptable for me to have a glass of
wine with dinner?

▼
TIP:

It may be. The key is the food you are eating. Alcohol can
cause severe, life-threatening low blood sugar, even in people who do not have diabetes. That is why we say drink only
with food. There is evidence that small amounts of alcohol are
okay for people with diabetes if they are not pregnant or do
not have a history of alcohol abuse. For example, one recent
study shows that moderate alcohol intake (no more than one
drink a day) is associated with lower blood sugar levels and
improved insulin sensitivity in healthy people who do not have
diabetes. Another study shows that blood sugar levels do not
differ for 12 hours after a meal between diabetic patients (both
types 1 and 2) who drink a shot of vodka before dinner, or a
glass of wine with dinner, or a shot of cognac after dinner and
those who drink an equal amount of water. Finally, a number
of studies have suggested that moderate alcohol intake may
have a positive effect on blood cholesterol and lipid levels. Just
remember that alcohol calories should be included in your
meal plan (one alcoholic drink is 1 fat exchange) and have
your one drink with food.

*H*ow can I reduce the
pain of frequent
finger sticks?

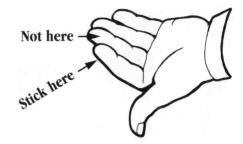

Not here →

Stick here →

▼
TIP:

O ne technique is to stick the side of your finger, where there are fewer pain sensors, instead of sticking directly into your fingerpad. Another technique is to use an automatic (spring-loaded) lancet holder that can vary how deep the lancet goes. Use the shortest depth that will give you an adequate drop of blood for testing. Since skin thickness varies from person to person, you'll need to try different depths to see what works for you.

Because of the danger of transmitting hepatitis and other blood-borne diseases, never "borrow" another person's device. Hopefully, in the next few years, noninvasive blood sugar monitors will become available for you to use. These monitors will sample your glucose level without having to stick your finger at all. In the meantime, there is a new lancet called Lancette that uses a laser to extract the drop of blood for testing. People who have tried it say that it is less painful to use. Talk with your health care team about this device and to get information on others that may be developed.

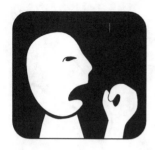

Why do I yawn when I have low blood sugar?

▼
TIP:

Probably because low blood sugar makes you feel tired. The classic signs and symptoms of low blood sugar include sweating, hunger, nervousness, and agitation. However, many people with diabetes do not have the usual symptoms. Some people have no symptoms at all!

Other people have unusual symptoms of low blood sugar. In some people, a change in their personality can occur; they become hostile and combative. Some people simply look "glassy-eyed," "spacey," or are mildly confused. It is very important to know what your low blood sugar symptoms are so that you know when to check it. And tell your friends and family so that they will know when to help you.

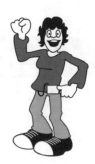

Would an insulin pump help me prevent complications?

▼
TIP:

Maybe. If it helps you keep your blood glucose close to normal levels, yes. But an insulin pump is not for everyone. If you have been unable to get your blood glucose levels into goal range, a pump may be a good choice for you. A pump, also called a "continuous subcutaneous insulin infusion system," can do some things that conventional insulin injection therapy can't. Using a pump requires motivation and a willingness to measure your blood sugar four or more times a day and to make decisions based on the results. A pump cannot "read" your blood sugar, so you have to do blood sugar tests regularly to tell the pump how much insulin you need. The downside is the cost. A pump costs about $5,000 to start and about $75 a month to maintain. You should talk to your health care team and insurance company about whether a pump would be a good idea for you. Newer pumps have more features and are more reliable than older models. More features allow more flexibility of lifestyle to help you stay in good control.

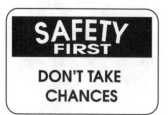

Is it safe for me to use birth control pills if I have diabetes?

▼
TIP:

Birth control pills appear to be safe for women with diabetes to take, and they are certainly safer than a pregnancy for which you are unprepared. There is controversy among diabetes specialists about the best form of birth control for women with diabetes. Under certain circumstances, estrogen-containing birth control pills may affect blood sugar and blood cholesterol levels. For this reason, some physicians have not prescribed them for women with diabetes. Studies have shown, however, that blood sugar levels are no different in women who take birth control pills than in women who do not. Similarly, blood cholesterol and lipid levels are no different in diabetic women who use birth control pills than in those who do not. There are other effective birth control methods, such as a diaphragm, that will not affect blood sugar at all. If you are concerned, talk to your health care team about which method of birth control will work best for you.

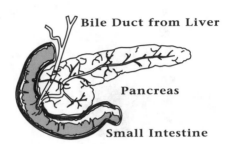

Would a successful pancreas transplant cure my diabetes?

▼
TIP:

Yes, but a pancreas transplant is not as easy as it sounds. Only a few hospitals in the United States do pancreas transplants. The problem with any transplant is rejection of the foreign tissue by our own bodies. There are drugs that suppress the body's rejection efforts, but these make diabetes control much more difficult. To be considered for a transplant, you have to meet criteria that may vary from center to center:

1. You must have type 1 diabetes.
2. Most centers will only do a pancreas transplant if you also need a kidney transplant. Antirejection drugs are expensive and hazardous, and the kidney transplant would automatically require the same antirejection drugs needed for the pancreas transplant.
3. You must have insurance or health coverage to pay for the transplant (many insurance programs consider this an experimental treatment and won't cover it), the medications, and the follow-up care needed after the transplant. A pancreas transplant may cost more than $100,000.

Perhaps we'll find new therapies to replace insulin-making cells without requiring antirejection medications.

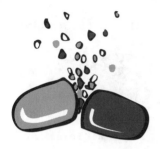

Why are my blood sugars high while I am taking prednisone for my asthma?

▼
TIP:

Prednisone is used for a variety of conditions such as asthma and other lung problems. It acts like a hormone that your body makes called "cortisol." Cortisol and prednisone both cause the body to make glucose when you're not eating (like during the night). They can worsen diabetes control. Cortisol is called a "stress hormone" because the body releases it to deal with stresses like accidents, infections, or burns. That's part of the reason why it takes more insulin to keep blood sugars near normal during an infection. If you have had prednisone prescribed for any reason and you have diabetes, you will need to take more diabetes medication. Prednisone's effect on your blood glucose will go away a day or two after you stop taking it. Your health care team can help you alter your diabetes treatment until you can stop taking the prednisone.

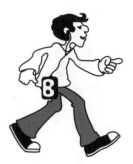

Will my 11-year-old son's diabetes have any long-term effects on his psychological health?

▼
TIP:

Coming to terms with a lifelong, chronic disease like diabetes is a big job for a child. It is not surprising that psychological problems can occur soon after diabetes develops. In general, most children who have family support adapt well and have no long-term psychological problems as a result.

One study has shown that children diagnosed with diabetes between the ages of 8 and 14 were initially more depressed, dependent, and socially withdrawn than other children. By the time a year had passed, most of these problems were gone. By 2 years after diagnosis, however, children with diabetes again had a higher risk of depression and dependency than children without diabetes.

Children seem to cope with the initial stress of developing diabetes, but as they realize that diabetes is a permanent condition, they may experience a period of depression. It is important for parents to realize this and to contact the health care team if you are concerned that your child might be depressed. In the interim, be supportive of your child and watchful for signs that might signal the onset of depression, such as a change in appetite, lack of interest in activities, or withdrawal from social groups.

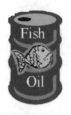

*A*re there any health benefits to fish oil?

▼
TIP:

Possibly. It is known that people with diabetes typically have elevated levels of fatty particles in their blood known as triglycerides. High levels of triglycerides are considered to be one of the reasons that people with diabetes have an increased risk for heart disease. Oils from a variety of fish, such as sardines, are thought to have beneficial effects on blood triglyceride concentrations in diabetic patients. A recent review of 26 separate studies concluded that fish oil may be of benefit in people who have diabetes and elevated triglyceride levels. Specifically, 2–5 teaspoons of fish oil were shown to reduce triglyceride levels by an average of 30–50%. Unfortunately, this was accompanied by a small increase in the levels of LDL cholesterol, another fatty particle that has been connected with the development of heart disease. Blood glucose levels may also be slightly increased by the daily use of fish oil. For now, you might consider replacing the red meat in your diet with fish several times a week. If you have high triglyceride levels, ask your doctor about the possibility of including a daily dose of fish oil.

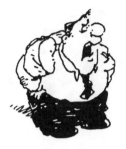

Why should I check my sugar when I can "feel" when it's high or low?

TIP:

Because you can't always feel it. Many people with diabetes believe that they have specific feelings when their sugar is either too high or too low. Although this may occasionally be true, it is unreliable. Studies have been done in people with diabetes in which their blood sugar has been acutely raised or lowered without them knowing which. They were then asked what they thought their blood sugar level was. No individual could accurately predict when his or her blood sugar was high or how high it was. On the other hand, many people could tell when their blood sugar was low or at least dropping rapidly. Unfortunately, when you consistently have high blood sugar, you often feel like your blood sugar is low even when it is still high. Because you make important decisions depending on your blood sugar level, always check your blood sugar before taking insulin, exercising, or driving a car.

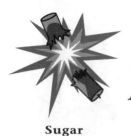

*H*ow can the sugar in my blood be
harmful when it's so common in food?

Sugar

▼
TIP:

The sugar in food is powerful. It can be thought of as tiny
packets of bundled-up energy. Normally, the body does
not let the amount of sugar in the blood rise very high because
it will react with the wrong tissues. In fact, of all the sub-
stances that circulate in your blood, sugar is one the body reg-
ulates most carefully. Even in people without diabetes, too
much sugar is thought to be responsible for many of the
changes that occur with aging. However, when a person has
diabetes, his or her body cannot prevent high blood glucose
levels from occurring. Over long periods of time, high levels
of sugar can cause serious damage to many tissues, especially
your eyes, kidneys, and nerves. This damage results in the
"complications" of diabetes. You can avoid or greatly delay
these complications by leading a healthy lifestyle and keeping
your blood sugar in your goal range.

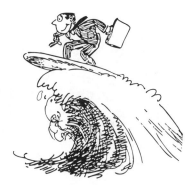

*S*hould I expect my blood sugars
to level off after I start a new
diabetes medicine?

TIP:

Y es. Blood sugars initially fall in response to the medicine.
But there is an effect that has to do with the fact that high
blood sugars tend to cause more high blood sugars. If your
blood sugar has been high for some time, your pancreas can't
immediately readjust. Your body has been using insulin poor-
ly. When you interrupt the cycle and spend more time in the
normal blood sugar range, you begin to increase your body's
ability to stay there. After several weeks of improved control,
many patients find that they need less insulin or oral medication to keep their blood sugars under control. It may take more
medication to get your blood sugars to begin to go down, but
how much medicine you need may decrease as your overall
diabetes control improves.

Some patients with type 2 diabetes who take a diabetes
medication and who also start exercising and eating better find
that, after a while, they can stop their medication as long as
they continue the other activities. Talk to your health care team
before stopping any medication. If you get the "go ahead,"
monitor your blood sugars while you continue with your diet
and exercise program. However, at the first sign that your
blood sugar levels are going back up, contact your team.

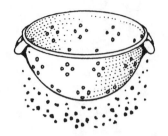

Why did my weight increase after I got my blood sugars under better control?

▼
TIP:

Some oral diabetes medications, such as glipizide and glyburide, and insulin will tend to cause weight gain when you achieve better blood sugar control. You are having a very common experience. When your blood sugars were high, you were losing many calories in your urine. The kidneys can only absorb a limited amount of sugar, and then, like a sieve, they let the extra sugar go through into the urine. This loss of sugar in the urine begins at a blood sugar level of about 200 mg/dl. So you waste part of the calories you are eating when your blood sugar exceeds this level. This may sound like a great way to eat too much and also control your weight, but the long-term effect of high sugar is very damaging to many parts of your body. Your body needs insulin to store amino acids (the building blocks of protein in muscle) and to make muscle. So, take your medication as prescribed by your health care team, reduce your food intake, and exercise regularly to control your weight.

Chapter 3
HEALTH FOODS

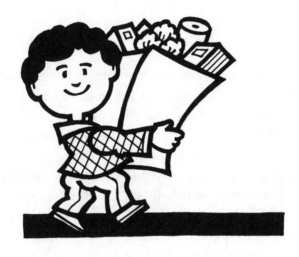

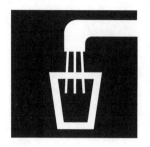

*Will chromium help me stay
healthy and improve my blood
sugar control?*

▼
TIP:

Your body does need some chromium to be healthy, but you're probably asking whether you need to take a chromium supplement. Most people do not need these supplements. Chromium is a naturally occurring mineral found in tap water and also present in tiny amounts in our bodies. Whether or not taking chromium will help you has been examined in many research studies. If you're getting enough chromium in your diet, there is no need for additional vitamin and mineral supplementation for most people with diabetes. Adequate diet means that you are getting a normal amount of calories from a variety of foods. Most people get into trouble when they eliminate one or more of the food groups or drastically reduce the calories needed to maintain a reasonable weight. Eat your fruits and vegetables, and don't go below 1,200 calories a day.

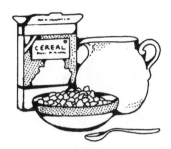

*W*ill fiber in my diet help me?

▼
TIP:

High-fiber foods may be beneficial to you, particularly if you have high blood fats or impaired glucose tolerance. Fiber is found primarily in fruits, vegetables, beans, and cereals, such as wheat and oats. Insoluble fibers like cellulose, found in wheat bran and celery, are dense and chewy. Soluble fibers, in whole oats and green peas, are soft and rather gel-like when mixed with water. Most fiber is not absorbed by the body, so it passes out in the stool. Any compounds that are bound by fiber in the intestine are also not absorbed. Many studies have been done to determine whether fiber is beneficial. Most studies show a positive (although limited) effect on blood fats. That's why high-fiber diets usually lower blood cholesterol. Some studies (primarily in type 2 diabetes) have also shown an improvement in blood sugar levels, but this improvement is usually small. You can add high-fiber foods, such as whole grains and beans, to your meals. Another way to increase the fiber in your diet is to take a tablespoon of pseudophilin (Metamucil) before you go to sleep.

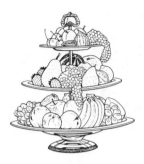

Should I use fructose as a sweetener when I bake?

▼
TIP:

Fructose is not necessarily better for you than plain sugar. Fructose is a naturally occurring sweetener like table sugar (sucrose). It may produce a smaller rise in blood sugar than the same number of calories of table sugar. This is good for people with diabetes; however, large amounts of fructose can increase your total cholesterol and "bad" cholesterol (LDL) levels. That's why fructose is really no better for you than other sugars. People with abnormal blood cholesterol levels should avoid consuming large amounts of fructose.

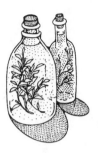

Will ginseng help me control my blood sugar?

▼
TIP:

Ginseng, derived from plants, is a chemical that has been used for many centuries to improve overall health and increase energy and well-being. It is often made into tea and taken with food. It is very popular in the U.S. and in some European and Asian countries. There are very few studies that test its beneficial effects in people with diabetes. Recently, one small short-term study from Finland suggested that individuals with type 2 diabetes who drink ginseng tea daily may have lower blood sugar levels than those who do not. Whether or not this effect lasts longer than 1 year is not known. At this time, ginseng is not a recommended treatment for diabetes, but that recommendation could change. Stay in touch with your health care team for updates.

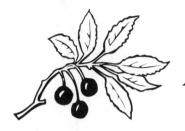

A re there any useful herbal remedies for diabetes?

▼
TIP:

We don't know. Diet or herbal remedies were all we had for most of the 2,000 years after diabetes was first described. Health food stores carry dozens of products designed for people with diabetes to use, ranging from blueberry leaf and wild cherry bark to preparations called "Hysugar" and "Losugar." Few of these products have been tested or proven to be safe and effective. Because herbal remedies are classified as food supplements, they are not regulated by the FDA. Moreover, none of these products alone result in adequate blood sugar control in most people with diabetes. You should discuss any antidiabetes health food products with your health care team. You may find that they are somewhat skeptical, but they will probably not object to the use of these products in moderation if you are demonstrating good control of your diabetes and doing the other things necessary to stay healthy with diabetes.

*W*hat is folic acid?

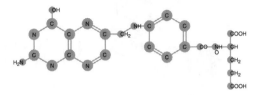

▼
TIP:

Folic acid (or folate) is a member of the B-vitamin family found in green, leafy vegetables. It plays an important role in several chemical processes in your body. Many medical experts are currently recommending that people increase their intake of folic acid because folic acid lowers homocysteine levels in our bodies. Homocysteine is a byproduct of the metabolic breakdown of a particular amino acid (the building blocks of proteins) called cysteine. There is a growing amount of scientific evidence suggesting that people with high levels of homocysteine are more likely to suffer from heart attacks or strokes. Although the issue remains to be settled, some studies suggest that people with diabetes have higher than normal amounts of homocysteine in their bodies, and this fact may be related to the increased number of heart attacks and strokes that occur in people with diabetes. Thus, it may be beneficial for people with diabetes to supplement their diet with the Recommended Daily Allowance (RDA) of 180–200 mcg per day for men and women and 400 mcg for pregnant women. This is the amount of folic acid usually found in daily multivitamin preparations.

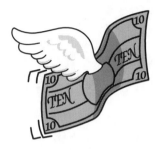

*W*ill *magnesium supplements help my diabetes?*

▼
TIP:

Probably not. The ADA does not recommend routine blood tests for magnesium levels, nor does it recommend that people take magnesium unless they have been shown to be deficient in this mineral. Magnesium deficiency may play a role in causing insulin resistance, carbohydrate intolerance, and high blood pressure. People who eat a varied diet probably won't become magnesium deficient because magnesium is found in many foods (including cereals, nuts, and green vegetables).

People at risk for magnesium deficiency are those with congestive heart failure, those with potassium or calcium deficiency, and those who are pregnant. Others at risk have had heart attacks, ketoacidosis, long-term feeding through the veins, long-term alcohol abuse, or have taken drugs such as diuretics over long periods of time. If a blood test shows these people need magnesium, a supplement may be given by the doctor. People with kidney disease should be very careful not to get too much magnesium and should only take it under a doctor's care.

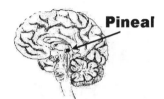

*I*s the melatonin miracle real?

▼
TIP:

There is very little scientific proof that taking melatonin supplements is beneficial. Melatonin is a substance that is normally secreted by a small part of the brain called the pineal gland. The exact role that it plays in humans is not clear, but research suggests that it may help regulate your sleep. It has become popular and is sold in health food stores. Many unproven beneficial effects have been attributed to melatonin, including better sleep, elimination of jet lag, reversal of the aging process, enhancement of sex, and protection against disease. Are these claims too good to be true? Yes. If you buy melatonin, you are probably just wasting your money. You may ask, "Is there any harm if I take melatonin for sleep?" The problem is that there are no long-term studies that show melatonin is safe. In fact, some doctors fear permanent damage to your normal sleep patterns if you take melatonin. There may also be other hazards that will become known only after melatonin has been in use several more years. For now, it is wise not to take melatonin supplements until there is better evidence to support its safety and effectiveness.

Chapter 4
NUTRITION ADVICE

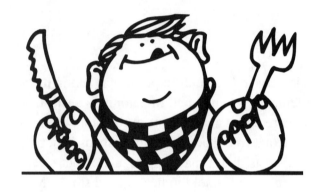

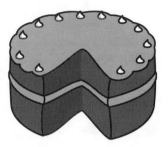

How can I overcome my craving for chocolate?

▼
TIP:

Give in once in a while! By denying your desire for chocolate (or any other particular food), you are setting yourself up for failure. If you find yourself craving a food and having to put effort into avoiding it, you may eventually give up and eat too much of it. Then your blood sugar control suffers, and you feel guilty and depressed. Think about some healthy ways to satisfy your craving. For chocolate lovers, dark or bitter chocolate is preferred to milk chocolate that has higher dairy fat. We suggest low-fat frozen yogurt. It tastes great, has less than 1 gram of fat, and is inexpensive. Another treat is chocolate graham crackers, which may also be used for making desserts. Make a fancy dessert with angel food cake, strawberries, and chocolate syrup. Yes, the syrup has some sugar in it, but it is almost fat free. Whether you have type 1 or type 2 diabetes, fat must be a concern for you and is actually the worst part of most candies. Recent research has shown that sugar has about the same effect as an equal amount of carbohydrate from potatoes or rice on your blood sugar. When you must have chocolate, substitute it into your meal plan for other carbohydrates. You can also look for some relatively low-fat chocolate foods that fit into your meal plan.

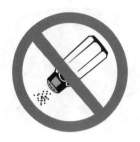

What diet change must I make to improve my blood pressure?

▼
TIP:

If you are sensitive to sodium, lowering the sodium in your diet may make a big difference in your blood pressure. Less sodium in your body means you will retain less water. There will be less fluid in your blood vessels and less "pressure" in the system. Sodium is a major part of table salt. Sodium is also used as a preservative and flavor enhancer in foods that may not even taste "salty." Try these tips to lower your sodium intake: 1) always taste your food before reaching for the salt shaker, 2) use pepper and other seasonings to add flavor before adding salt, 3) cook with a variety of seasonings or onion and garlic, 4) add a dash of lemon juice to vegetables and salads to brighten the flavor, 5) use garlic powder or fresh garlic instead of "seasoned salt" or garlic salt, 6) try a commercial salt-free seasoning mix and carry a small container with you, 7) ask for foods to be prepared without salt in restaurants and ask for sauces "on the side", 8) read the labels on prepared foods and canned goods to find the high-salt items and look for no-salt-added or low-sodium products.

Remember, the closer to nature a food is, the more likely it will be low in sodium.

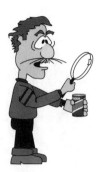

Can reading food labels help me stay healthy?

▼
TIP:

Yes. Food labels give you important information that can help you eat healthy meals and snacks. New regulations by the FDA have increased the information that must be put on food labels. Food labels must include

1. The standard serving size
2. Calories and calories from fat in each serving
3. A list of nutrients and ingredients
4. The recommended daily amounts of nutrients in the food
5. The relationship between the food and any disease it may affect

Try to make a habit of reading the labels of the foods you buy and become familiar with the amount of calories, fat, carbohydrate, and sodium in them. For many foods, you will have a choice of different brand names, and by comparing the information on the labels, you can choose the brand that is healthier. Food label information helps you keep track of the amount of nutrients that you are eating daily. This information is vital to a healthy diet.

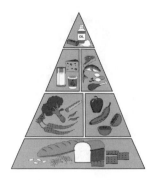

*W*ill the USDA Food Guide
Pyramid help me live healthier
with diabetes?

▼
TIP:

Yes. The food guide pyramid was developed as a guide to
healthy eating for all Americans. It's healthy eating for
people with diabetes, too. The pyramid shape tells you how
much to eat of different foods. The bottom section—the largest
section—is the bread, cereal, rice, and pasta group, and most
people should eat 6–11 servings a day. The two sections above
starches are vegetables (3–5 servings a day) and fruits (2–4
servings a day). These first three sections together cover more
than half of the pyramid. This tells you that half or more of
your daily food intake should come from these foods. The next
two sections are the dairy (2–3 servings a day) and the meat,
poultry, and fish group (2–3 servings a day). You don't need as
much of these foods. Also, they may be high in fat. The small
top section contains the fats, oils, and sweets group. You need
very little of these foods, which is why they don't have serving
suggestions. They can be very high in calories without much
nutrition. Following the food guide pyramid can be an easy
and healthy way for a person with diabetes to achieve good
health and nutrition. ADA has developed a Diabetes Food
Pyramid that is very similar to the USDA pyramid. Ask your
RD for help using these nutrition tools.

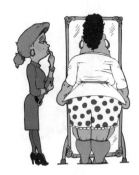

Should I join an expensive diet and weight-reduction program to lose weight?

▼
TIP:

We don't recommend it. You will probably waste your time and your money. Advertisements for these programs usually show "before" and "after" photographs of heavy people who have lost weight. What these advertisements don't show you are the people who never lost a pound. More importantly, long-term studies have shown that almost all of the people who lose weight rapidly over several months gain it all back by the end of 5 years. This has also been the experience of our patients who have tried these programs. Also, very-low-calorie diets (VLCDs) can be dangerous because they can cause serious chemical imbalances and vitamin deficiencies. A much better plan to lose weight is to make small changes in your lifestyle so that you lose only 1/2–1 pound per month. Over 5 years, this small change equals a 50-pound weight loss! In comparison to expensive diet programs, low cost weight-reduction programs, such as Weight Watchers or TOPS (Take Off Pounds Sensibly), can provide much support and advice for you. In addition, your health care team can be of great help in suggesting ways of making small but positive changes in your lifestyle to accomplish your weight goals.

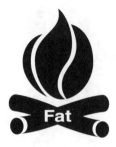

Why do I spill ketones in my urine?

TIP:

Ketones in the urine show that fat is being burned for fuel by your body. This typically occurs when you do not have enough insulin in your body to metabolize sugar as fuel or when you are fasting (dieting or not eating because you are sick). Thus, spilling ketones into your urine means either that your body is dangerously low on insulin or that your diet is working. When ketones build up because of a lack of insulin, the condition is called "ketoacidosis," and it can be dangerous. Ketoacidosis is more common in type 1 diabetes and occurs when people first develop diabetes, when they stop taking insulin for some reason, or when they are ill. Most people develop symptoms that make them consult a doctor, such as stomach pain, nausea or vomiting, rapid breathing, frequent urination, extreme thirst, or fatigue.

If you are on a diet that does not provide enough calories to your body, then your body burns fat for energy. This is the effect you want from your diet, because burning fat will cause you to lose weight. A by-product of fat metabolism, however, is ketones, and these ketones spill into your urine just as they do in ketoacidosis. If you are feeling fine and controlling your blood sugar, then the ketones in your urine are probably a safe result of your diet.

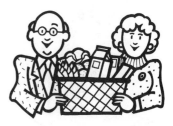

How can I get my spouse to follow his/her meal plan?

▼
TIP:

We have several suggestions. There are many reasons why your spouse might not follow the prescribed meal plan. First, s/he may not understand it. Did s/he see an RD and receive easily understood written instructions describing the meal plan? Second, your spouse may not believe that following it will work. Ask him/her to try the prescribed plan for 1 month and measure weight and blood sugar daily to see what the effects are. Then s/he can decide whether the meal plan will help achieve his/her goals. Third, your spouse may not want to eat foods that are "different" from those that the rest of the family eats. It helps if the whole family changes to a healthier diet. (A meal plan is the same balanced healthy diet that everyone should eat.) The RD can help him/her fit some of his/her favorite foods into the meal plan. Fourth, do you understand the details of the plan? If you select and prepare the food that your spouse eats, you may want to discuss the meal plan with your RD. Finally, remember that changing eating habits will involve a change in lifestyle, which is difficult for anyone. Don't try to change too many things too quickly. Your spouse will need support, understanding, and patience to achieve his/her goals.

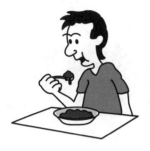

*I*s it a good idea to eat four or five
small meals during the day instead
of three large meals?

▼
TIP:

Y es! Scientists have been looking for the ideal frequency of
meals since the beginning of diabetes research. There are
many benefits to eating small amounts of food over the course
of the day instead of larger amounts at meal times. These benefits include decreased blood sugar levels after a meal, reduced
insulin requirements over the course of the day, and decreased
blood cholesterol levels. These benefits probably stem from a
slow, continuous absorption of food from your gut, which
spares your body the work of switching over to a "fasting"
state. Also, eating several small meals a day may decrease your
hunger and reduce the number of calories you eat during the
day. Finally, there are diabetes medications available, such as
acarbose, that slow the absorption of food and have much the
same effect as eating your food slowly over the course of the
day. The practice of nibbling is not for everyone; but if it helps
you maintain good blood sugar control and a desirable body
weight when doing it, then continue.

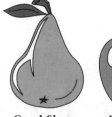

*H*ow can I use the waist/hip *ratio to improve my health?*

Good Shape **Bad Shape**

▼
TIP:

The waist/hip ratio can be used to predict your risk of developing heart disease in the future. Take a tape measure and measure the circumference of your body at its largest diameter at the level of your hips. Next, measure the size of your waist (your stomach) at its largest diameter. Be honest, don't pull in your stomach when measuring. Okay, now you are ready. Divide your waist size in inches by your hip size in inches. If the answer is less than 1.0 for men (or 0.85 for women), then your shape is good. What this means is that your body is pear shaped rather than apple shaped. If the result is more than 1.0 for men (or 0.85 for women), you are at an increased risk of developing heart disease. The reason for the increased risk is that you have more fat in the stomach area than on your hips and thighs. For unknown reasons, fat located above the hips is a major risk factor for future heart disease. If you are at an increased risk and overweight, you need to work on losing weight. After you have lost 5 pounds, you could remeasure your waist/hip ratio. Ideally you want to reduce your weight until your waist/hip ratio is below 1.0 if you are a man (0.85 if you are a woman). All obesity is bad for your health, but obesity above your waist is especially hazardous.

Chapter 5
COMPLICATIONS—MICRO*

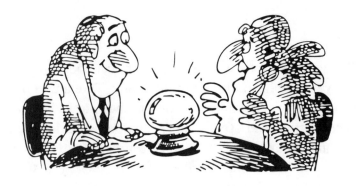

*disease of the small blood vessels

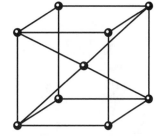

*W*hat does the term AGE mean in
reference to diabetes?

TIP:

Good question! AGE is an abbreviation for advanced glyco-
sylation end product. This complicated name describes
the process of sugar becoming permanently attached to body
tissues. The sugar may cause damage such that the tissues can
no longer carry out their normal function.

A common example is glycosylated (glycated) hemoglobin,
which is glucose permanently attached to hemoglobin protein
in your red blood cells. However, since new red blood cells are
continuously made by your body, little long-term damage
results from this attached glucose. In contrast, tissues in your
eyes, kidneys, and nerves remain in your body for a long period
of time, so the attached sugar can do significant damage.

A new medicine called aminoguanidine can block sugar
from permanently attaching to and damaging your body
tissues. Hopefully, this medicine will prevent some of the
complications of diabetes. This medicine is currently being
tested in many medical centers throughout the United States.
Studies in animals suggest it should work well in humans. If it
does, then many of the complications of diabetes will be
preventable.

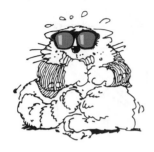

What kinds of eye problems are caused by diabetes?

▼
TIP:

Diabetes is the number one cause of blindness in the United States. Fortunately, many eye problems are treatable if they are identified early. One of the most serious eye problems caused by diabetes is retinopathy. In this disease, fragile blood vessels grow in the back of the eye and can bleed easily. Such bleeding can cloud the vision and lead to permanent scarring of the back of the eye (the retina). People with diabetes may also have cataracts (a permanent clouding of the lens), "floaters" that temporarily interfere with vision, and a swelling of the eye nerves that can cause permanent damage to your sight (macular edema). Abnormal function of the nerves that control the eye muscles can result in double vision. All people who develop double vision should see an eye doctor as soon as possible to rule out other possible causes, such as a small stroke. Cataracts can be corrected surgically. Laser therapy helps stop retinopathy or macular edema if it is performed before there is too much damage. A yearly eye examination by a doctor who specializes in diabetic eye disease is the best way to detect eye problems in the early stages, and keeping your blood sugar near normal can help reduce your risk of eye disease.

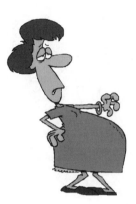

*W*hy would my health care team be
concerned about my becoming
*pregnant if I have high blood pressure and
have had laser treatment of my eye
problems?*

TIP:

Many changes in blood flow and pressure occur during
pregnancy that can aggravate eye disease and kidney disease. The number of blood pressure medications that can be
used safely during pregnancy and not injure a developing fetus
are limited. You should discuss the options and the severity of
your complications openly with your health care team as part
of your pre-pregnancy planning process. Existing complications of diabetes can get worse during pregnancy. This is not to
say that you should not get pregnant if you have mild diabetic
complications. Many women with long-standing diabetes are
able to have a normal pregnancy. However, the complications
may make the pregnancy more difficult. One means of assess-
ing the risks of pregnancy is called the "White classification,"
named for Dr. Priscilla White, the physician who developed it.
It is used by some obstetricians specializing in patients with
diabetes. The length of time that you have had diabetes and the
severity of your complications will determine your level of risk
in the White classification.

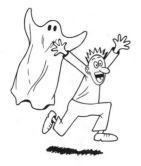

*C*an I ignore the risks of diabetic complications, since the thought of them scares me?

▼
TIP:

No, because there are some things you can do now to prevent the disabling complications of diabetes. Adjusting your food, physical activity, and medication (if any) to bring your blood glucose levels to near-normal ranges can help you avoid or delay complications. Research has proven that. You are expressing emotions that most of us go through at some time in our lives. All of us have fears of growing old or disabled, whether we have diabetes or not. The challenge we all face is how to live a healthy life. We all want to live well every day that we live. We want to be fully functional and independent. You can decide to ignore the changes taking place in your body, but that won't make them go away. Or you can take charge to change the outcome so that you can live your life without fear. Your knowledge of the effects of diabetic complications on your body is information that can give you power over the future!

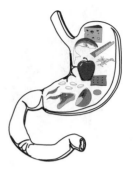

*D*uring a meal, why do I get filled up
before I finish eating?

▼
TIP:

Your symptoms may be caused by a complication of diabetes
called "diabetic gastroparesis." It means that the stomach
empties very slowly. It is caused by damage to the nerves that
control the pace at which food leaves the stomach and gets
processed in the gut. Some people experience nausea, while
others may only note that they can't eat as much at one time.
If the rate of food emptying from your stomach is too slow and
you took insulin before the meal, your blood sugar may fall
before the food has had a chance to be absorbed. You may
have to adjust when you take your insulin injection or oral
medication to prevent low blood sugars and to match the
absorption of carbohydrate from your meal. High-fiber or
high-fat foods tend to make gastroparesis worse. There are
some medications that can help improve gut function. Talk to
your health care team about the best approach for you.

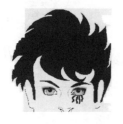

*C*ould my diabetes cause one of
my eyes to be red and painful?

▼
TIP:

Perhaps. Allergies to pollens and dust in the air are the most common cause of red eyes, but they rarely cause pain. An eye infection that can cause red eyes is viral conjunctivitis, or "pink eye." Unfortunately, this infection has to run its course because antibiotics cannot help speed recovery. Serious bacterial infections can start on the surface of or behind the eye of a person with diabetes and require strong antibiotics to cure. A common complaint of patients with either viral or bacterial infections is that they wake up in the morning with their eyelashes sticking together from the pus that has collected over the night.

If your pain is more like a pressure sensation, then you may have glaucoma. Glaucoma is too much pressure in the eye and is more common in people with diabetes. It can be detected during your yearly eye exam. The test involves blowing a small puff of air (which doesn't hurt) at the surface of the eye. Your doctor may prescribe eye drops that lower the pressure in the eye. This condition is definitely worth finding early because it is treatable. Left untreated, glaucoma can result in blindness.

*W*ill my diabetic kidney disease get
worse if I get pregnant?

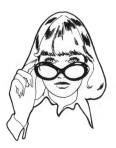

▼
TIP:

There is about a 30% chance that your kidney function will worsen during pregnancy, but these changes often improve after delivery of the infant. Many women with diabetes will first show signs of abnormal kidney function (spilling protein into the urine) during pregnancy. If you have kidney disease before getting pregnant, then there is a chance that it will get worse during pregnancy.

Moreover, babies born to mothers with diabetic kidney disease have a higher risk of stillbirth, respiratory distress, jaundice, and abnormally small body size compared to babies of diabetic mothers without kidney problems. Also, about 30% of these babies are born prematurely. You will need to have tight blood sugar control and careful control of blood pressure before and during the pregnancy. It takes hard work to maintain near-normal blood sugars throughout a pregnancy, but it is necessary for your health and the baby's. You should know the risks before you get pregnant.

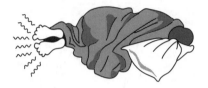

*W*hy do my feet burn at night when I'm trying to go to sleep?

▼
TIP:

The nerves in your feet have been affected by your diabetes. "Painful neuropathy" is a term used to describe pain without an obvious cause. People with painful neuropathy usually describe a "pins and needles" sensation or a dull burning in the feet and legs that is more apparent at night (when there are few other things to distract you). You may also experience frequent leg cramps. Because painful neuropathy is difficult to cure once it is established, the best treatment is to prevent it by controlling your blood sugar. These nerve problems occur more frequently in men and in people who have had diabetes for many years, are tall, smoke, or have poor blood sugar control.

If you already have painful neuropathy, there are treatments available that provide some relief for about 50% of people. These treatments include the use of antidepressant medicines, certain heart medications, medications such as Dilantin and Tegretol, and creams made from chili peppers (capsaicin). These creams are rubbed on the feet to desensitize them. If you do not get relief from one of these treatments, the good news is that the pain from this neuropathy often lessens over time.

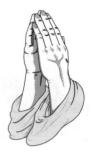

*I*s there a simple test to see whether my
diabetes is causing my hands to be stiff
and rigid?

▼
TIP:

High blood sugars over a long period of time can increase
the stiffness of tissue around your finger joints. This can
eventually cause stiff hands and prevent you from straightening
your fingers. This stiffness may make it difficult to write or to
pick up small items and do other fine movements. An easy test
for this condition is called the "prayer sign," in which you hold
your hands together, one palm facing the other palm, to see
whether your fingers can lie flat against each other. If a space
exists between your right and left hands when you try to push
your hands together (as in the above figure), this is a "positive" prayer sign. High sugars may be causing this condition.
Arthritis can also cause a positive prayer sign. In the near
future, new medications may become available that will reduce
this stiffness. In the meantime, you should try to keep your
blood sugars as close to your goal range as possible.

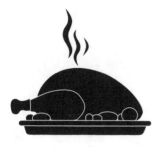

S hould I eat more protein to replace the protein I am losing in my urine?

▼
TIP:

U sually the answer is no. The protein that you are losing in your urine (known as "spilling protein") is a sign that the filters in your kidney are showing wear and tear. Normally, the blood in your body goes through your kidneys to remove waste products. Kidneys act like a sieve that retains valuable chemicals but lets water go through. The protein in your blood is supposed to stay in your body, but when the kidney filters are damaged from years of high blood sugar and high blood pressure, they let protein slip through as well. Also, the waste products from protein can be stressful to the kidney.

Reducing the amount of protein in your diet may help the kidneys and slow damage to them. You should talk to your health care provider or RD about reducing protein in your diet. You might not know that many foods such as cereals and grains contain protein. You may need help designing a meal plan that helps you reduce overall protein but gives you the essential types and amounts that you need. Wise food choices and following your meal plan are an important part of keeping your kidneys healthy.

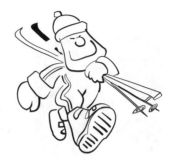

Should I limit my exercise program for 1 month after laser therapy on my eyes?

TIP:

Yes. Diabetic eye disease (retinopathy) is a condition of overgrowth of fragile blood vessels in the eye that can cause bleeding, scarring, and loss of vision if they break. Even though you have had laser therapy, you should still be careful to avoid situations that can stress these vessels. Avoid exercises that cause you to strain, such as weight lifting or any exercise that causes you to hold your breath. Underwater diving can also cause increased pressure in the eye and should be avoided. Another consequence of laser therapy is the possibility of a loss in peripheral vision (the ability to see clearly off to the side). For this reason, some sports (such as racquetball or tennis) may be hazardous because they require you to respond to a ball coming at a high speed from all angles. You should discuss any exercise program with your eye doctor if you have had laser therapy.

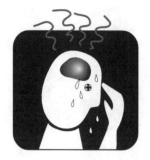

Why have I recently begun to sweat profusely when I sit down and eat food, even though the food does not contain hot, spicy items?

▼
TIP:

One complication of diabetes that is related to nerve damage is called "gustatory sweating." The person with diabetes breaks out in a sweat from chewing food. The cause of this sweating is not known, but it may be related to having high blood sugars for a long time. You may also have increased sweating or flushing of the neck and chest. Cheese and chocolate are the most common foods to cause sweating, but pickles, alcohol, vinegar, fresh fruits, and salty foods may do it, too. Various types of medications have been tried to treat this problem, with varying levels of success. Although in some cases it stops by itself, try to keep your blood sugar as normal as possible and avoid specific foods that may cause sweating.

Chapter 6
COMPLICATIONS—MACRO*

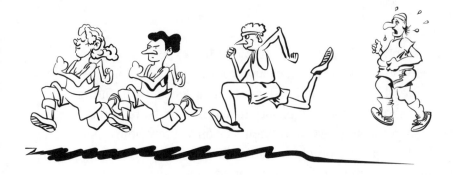

*disease of the large blood vessels

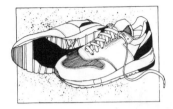

I don't want to end up with foot problems; how do I know whether my athletic shoes are okay?

▼
TIP:

It is best to buy shoes from a store that has experienced personnel who know how to measure your feet and fit your shoes correctly. A "certified pedorthist" is a specialist in fitting shoes and shoe inserts for a proper fit with no pressure points. When you get new shoes, wear them for only a few hours, and then check your feet for any red areas or sore places where the shoes might be rubbing. Even well-fitted shoes may have a seam or an area that rubs on your foot. Get padded athletic socks that protect your feet from blisters. Athletic shoes have become very high-tech these days and have different features depending on the exercise you are planning to do. It is a good idea to get the ones with extra cushion because this reduces the wear and tear on your joints. Look in the Yellow Pages for stores that specialize in athletic shoes or have a pedorthist on staff.

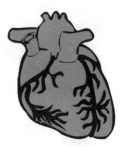

*A*m I at more risk of developing heart
disease because I have diabetes?

▼
TIP:

Yes. For unknown reasons, having diabetes does put you at
an increased risk for heart disease and other diseases that
are caused by blocked arteries. In fact, your risk is the same as
a person without diabetes who has already had one heart attack.
That is why it is very important for you to minimize your other
risk factors by getting plenty of exercise, keeping your weight
normal, avoiding cholesterol and fatty foods (saturated fat),
and maintaining normal blood pressure. Walking is a good
exercise and helps in all those areas as well as in reducing
stress. Most important (at least in our opinion) is that you do not
smoke cigarettes. If you are already smoking, join a "quit smoking" support group. These are available in most communities
and health care facilities. Nicotine skin patches may help.
Many of the risk factors that contribute to heart disease can be
greatly reduced with a healthy lifestyle, and this should be
your goal with or without diabetes. However, because you
already have one risk factor for heart disease (diabetes), there
is even more reason to reduce other risk factors.

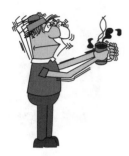

*W*hy do I get dizzy when I stand up?

▼
TIP:

Patients with long-term diabetes may lose the ability to maintain their blood pressure in response to changes in posture. Your blood pressure may drop very low when you stand up and cause dizziness, temporary loss of vision, or fainting spells.

You may be experiencing "postural dizziness," which can be serious. Abnormal function of the nerves that regulate your heart and blood vessels is the most common cause of postural dizziness, but other causes must be ruled out by your health care team. Blood pressure medications, such as diuretics, can cause postural dizziness and so can antidepressants, nitroglycerine, and certain calcium-blocking drugs.

If your postural dizziness is due to diabetes alone, then you will need specific treatment for this problem. Tilting your bed so that the head is 6–9 inches higher than the foot may reduce your dizziness when you get up. Other therapies include carefully increasing the salt in your diet, wearing support stockings to prevent blood from pooling in your legs, or taking a hormone pill (Florinef) to help your body retain fluid. These treatments can be dangerous in people who have heart disease, so be sure to consult your health care team before trying any of them.

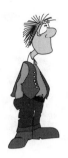

*I*s my 25 years of diabetes to blame for
my recent trouble maintaining erections?

▼
TIP:

Maybe, but there are other causes for this condition. Your
doctor should begin by checking for psychological and
emotional causes. This includes asking you questions about
depression, because depression affects sex drive. Other causes
may be poor circulation to the penis or low hormone levels.
Blood flow to the penis may be too low to get or maintain
erections. Long-term high blood sugars can affect these blood
vessels or the nerves to the penis. If this is the problem, there
are devices to aid you in getting an erection. All men have
reduced male hormone levels as they get older. Replacing
these hormones with monthly injections (or daily skin patches)
of testosterone may improve sex drive. There is an oral medication that helps up to 60% of men with diabetes obtain erections
(Viagra). This medication has proven very popular but is
expensive. Some high blood pressure medications can cause
sexual problems as a side effect, and switching from one to
another may help. Drinking alcohol can affect male hormone
levels and can depress your brain's ability to get sexually
aroused. There are many causes and many treatments for erectile
dysfunction. See your health care team for an evaluation or
referral to a specialist.

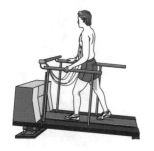

Should I have a yearly test to see if I have heart disease?

▼
TIP:

Ask your diabetes care team each year if you have any health complaints that would indicate that a heart test is necessary. Heart disease is the cause of death in about 80% of people with diabetes. People with diabetes do not always develop symptoms (such as chest pain) when they are having heart stress or even a heart attack, and heart disease can occur at a young age. Testing is required to diagnose heart disease at a stage when it is treatable. If you have had diabetes for many years, ask your health care team whether a screening test for silent heart disease is necessary—especially if you plan to start an exercise program or you have multiple risks for developing heart disease. Your health care team will probably refer you to a heart doctor (cardiologist) for these tests, and the type of tests may vary. Some cardiologists prefer a simple exercise treadmill test, in which your heart is monitored while you walk uphill on a treadmill. Many cardiologists now prefer to stress your heart with a medication instead of exercise. A test, called a dipyridamole stress test, shows how your heart functions when it works hard and may reveal areas of heart damage. This damage may then be treated with medications or surgery.

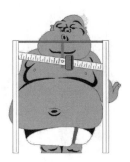

*S*ince I can't reach or see my toes very
well, how can I adequately care for
my feet?

▼
TIP:

Many people with diabetes have difficulty seeing their feet
well and trimming their toenails. The reasons for this
problem are many, including poor eyesight, obesity, arthritis,
back pain, and other medical conditions that may prevent you
from leaning over toward the floor. Have a member of your
family or a friend examine your feet once a day for sores and
nail problems. We strongly recommend that most people with
diabetes do not try to cut their own toenails, but go regularly to
a podiatrist for routine foot care. Podiatrists are trained to provide good foot hygiene and nail care. They can be located in
the Yellow Pages under Physicians & Surgeons, DPM (Podi-
atric), or you can ask your health care team for a referral.
Good foot care is extremely important to your good health. It
may save your feet.

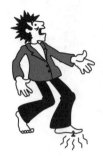

*D*o I need to have special foot care if my feet don't hurt?

TIP:

Yes. If you have had diabetes for many years, it is common not to feel pain in your feet. Thus, you may not notice sores and blisters that would normally cause you to avoid walking. Even if you don't have any sores, corns, calluses, or thickened toenails, you should still check your feet daily and use a moisturizing lotion after bathing—but not between your toes. Going barefoot is not recommended because of possible injuries to your bare feet. Always take off your shoes and socks during your quarterly visit to the health care team as a reminder to have your feet checked. The team will test to see whether you can feel a soft touch or have little changes of direction in your toes, and they will examine your reflexes and your ability to feel a tuning fork vibration. They will look for areas of skin breakdown on the bottom of your feet and between your toes and will check to be sure that you do not have an ingrown toenail. Ingrown nails easily become infected and require special care. You should see a podiatrist if you have a tendency to develop ingrown toenails. A podiatrist will also remove any calluses that you have. Many of the infections that end in leg amputation start out as tiny, nonpainful foot sores that don't heal.

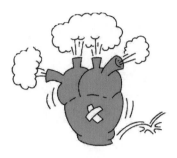

*W*hy *did my doctor start me on a cholesterol-lowering drug even though my cholesterol levels are only borderline high?*

▼
TIP:

Because your doctor wants to prevent or delay heart disease. Heart disease is the number one cause of death in people with diabetes. The levels of fats (cholesterol and triglycerides) in your blood are one of the most important ways to determine your risk for developing heart disease. People with diabetes tend to develop heart disease with lower lipid levels than nondiabetic patients, so some doctors try early on to lower blood lipid levels in their diabetic patients. This is probably a good idea, especially if you are a person who has several other risk factors for the development of heart disease. These risk factors include smoking, high blood pressure, and a history of heart disease at a young age among your close family members.

Because the risk of heart disease is high among all people with diabetes, they should stop smoking, eat a low-fat and low-cholesterol diet, avoid weight gain, and exercise regularly. If these measures fail to lower blood fat levels, then drug therapy is usually considered.

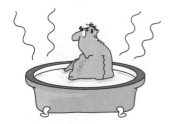

If I am on insulin, is it all right for me to sit in a hot tub?

▼
TIP:

Under certain conditions. People with diabetes should be careful with hot tubs and saunas. Excessive heat can make your heart beat faster, and if you have an underlying heart problem (like angina), you may end up with serious heart damage. When your whole body gets overheated, your heart tries to increase the blood flow to your skin to get rid of some of the extra heat you have absorbed from the water or steam. If you use insulin to control your diabetes, you may find that this increased blood flow to the fat (where you inject your insulin) increases the rate at which the insulin is absorbed. So a dose of a longer-acting insulin that is intended to last throughout the night will be absorbed much more rapidly. This causes low blood sugars during the hours after you get out of the tub. We recommend temperatures no higher than 105° and that you stay in the water for no longer than 20 minutes. Discuss your plans with your health care team.

*W*hy do I sometimes leak urine?

▼
TIP:

Approximately 25% of all people with long-term diabetes have some problems with bladder function. Most of these problems result from faulty signals from the nerves that control the bladder. Some of these problems are minor, such as an inability to empty your bladder completely when you urinate, a slow rate of urine flow, or an inability to tell when your bladder is full until it is overflowing. When you accidentally leak urine, the problem is usually more advanced and is called "incontinence." The most common cause of incontinence is an inability to tell whether your bladder is full, so the bladder becomes too full and overflows. Men with incontinence often have an enlarged prostate gland pressing on the bladder, and this can be treated with medicine or corrected by surgery. All men with diabetes over the age of 40 should have a prostate exam every year. If you have overflow incontinence, you may be able to manage the problem by reminding yourself to urinate on a schedule every day. You may strengthen the muscles around the bladder by doing "kegel" exercises (tensing and relaxing) or stopping the flow of urine several times. If you continue to have trouble, seek help from a bladder specialist (a urologist).

*W*ill lowering the fat in my diet reduce my risk for heart disease?

Type of fat	Effect on your body	In summary...
Saturated fat: animal fats, lard	increases cholesterol; increases heart disease	☹
Monounsaturated fat: olive oil, canola oil, nuts, avocado	lowers cholesterol; no effect on HDL ("good" cholesterol)	☺
Polyunsaturated fat: corn oil, safflower oil	lowers cholestero;l positive and negative effect on HDL	☺

▼
TIP:

In most cases, yes. You will especially lower your risk if you lower the saturated fats. Fats fall into one of three groups. **Saturated fats** increase cholesterol in your blood and, therefore, the risk of heart disease. They are usually solid at room temperature and are found in animal fats (meat, butter, lard, bacon, cheese), coconut, palm, and palm kernel oils, dairy fats, and hydrogenated vegetable fats (such as vegetable shortening and stick margarine).

Monounsaturated fats lower total cholesterol, do not affect HDL levels, and may reduce triglyceride levels. Food sources are olive oil, peanut oil, canola oil, olives, avocados, and nuts (except walnuts, which are polyunsaturated).

Polyunsaturated fats lower cholesterol levels but may also lower HDL levels. Food sources are vegetable oils such as corn, safflower, soybean, sunflower, and cottonseed.

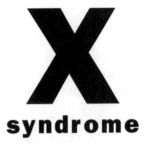

syndrome

Is my high blood pressure related to my diabetes?

▼
TIP:

Probably. People with diabetes are more likely to have high blood pressure. And people with the following symptoms are more likely to develop diabetes or heart disease. The combination of high blood pressure, high blood fat levels (triglycerides), obesity (primarily around and above the waist), and insulin resistance is commonly called "syndrome X." It is not a specific disease but a group of related risk factors that often exist together. A person with syndrome X is at a higher risk of developing diabetes and heart disease. Syndrome X is very common and may affect up to 25% of all middle-aged American males (and less commonly, females). So, to answer your question, high blood pressure and diabetes are related and often occur in the same individual. The important health message is that a person with syndrome X should immediately seek medical advice to reduce his or her weight and blood pressure. You should not wait until you develop diabetes or heart disease to change to a healthier lifestyle.

Chapter 7
MISCELLANEOUS

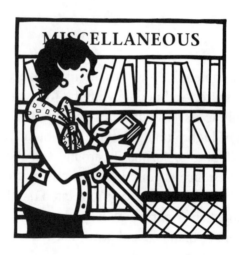

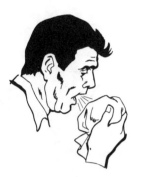

What can I take for a cough that is caused by my ACE inhibitor medication?

▼
TIP:

Many people with diabetes have problems with high blood pressure. Angiotensin-converting enzyme (ACE) inhibitors are ideal medications for this problem. One of their side benefits is to reduce blood pressure in the kidneys and to protect them from damage. Studies have shown that these medications actually reduce the rate of kidney damage caused by diabetes. Unfortunately, these drugs also affect the lungs, and about 20% of people treated with them develop an annoying cough. Although this cough is not dangerous, some patients have to stop taking their ACE inhibitor medication because they can't tolerate the cough. Losartan (Cozaar), a new type of ACE inhibitor, has recently been approved by the FDA. This drug has many of the benefits of the other ACE inhibitors on your blood pressure and kidneys, but it does not cause a cough. Ask your health care team whether this might be a good medication for you.

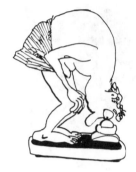

Why do I gain weight as I get older?

▼
TIP:

Unfortunately, most people do gain weight as they get older. There are several reasons. As you get older, your activity level changes to less strenuous exercise. For example, in the 20- to 30-year-old age group, many people jog, play tennis, work out at health clubs, etc. In later years, people change activities to include golf, bowling, and watching television. As your activities change, you burn fewer calories. If you're still eating the same amount of food that you always have, weight gain will follow. In addition, recent studies have suggested that older people are actually more efficient at storing food as fat. This means that for the same amount of food eaten, more exercise is needed to use it up. You should gradually decrease the amount of food that you eat as you get older to keep your body weight normal. In general, the leaner you are, the longer you will live.

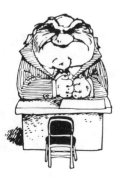

*C*an my diabetes cause constipation?

▼
TIP:

Yes. Constipation is the most common gastrointestinal disorder in people with diabetes, affecting about one in four patients. Your chances of having constipation increase to 50% if you have nerve problems due to diabetes. Most episodes of constipation in people with diabetes are caused by failure of the nerves that control the muscles of the bowel or large intestine to work properly. Other possible causes include blockage by a large amount of hard, dry stool; low levels of thyroid hormone; or an undiagnosed tumor. If you have frequent problems, you should ask your health care team for a complete evaluation of your bowel, including thyroid hormone tests. This evaluation may include a diagnostic test called a barium enema or a procedure in which a stomach and intestinal specialist (gastroenterologist) inspects your bowel with a fiber-optic viewing device (a colonoscope). If it turns out that your constipation is caused by diabetes alone, then you may get relief by adding fiber to your diet or a gentle laxative, such as docusate.

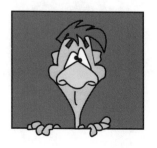

Should I be concerned about a blood pressure of 128/86 mmHg?

▼
TIP:

The most recent American Heart Association guidelines suggest that diastolic blood pressure (the bottom number) above 85 puts you at increased risk. Even mild elevations in blood pressure like yours increase the risk of complications such as retinopathy (eye disease), nephropathy (kidney disease), and heart disease. You should discuss these readings with your health care team. If your blood pressure readings are consistently high, you may need to start on blood pressure medication. Your doctor may ask you to check your blood pressure many times and in different settings to determine whether your blood pressure is high all the time or goes up only at specific times. If you haven't tried using exercise and nutrition to decrease your blood pressure, it's time to start a walking program and to decrease the sodium in your diet. The recommended amount of sodium is 2,400 mg per day or less. Start by taking the salt shaker off the table. Read labels on foods to identify (and then reduce) the high-sodium foods in your diet. Canned goods and processed foods may be high in sodium. Drinking alcohol can also raise your blood pressure.

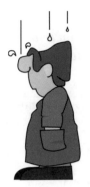

*H*ow do I handle the depression of having had diabetes for 25 years?

▼
TIP:

Depression is a common condition in people with chronic diseases like diabetes. Recognizing the symptoms of depression and making the diagnosis are keys to treating it. A lack of energy, changes in eating habits, changes in sleep patterns (sleep disturbances that may lead to daytime drowsiness), and loss of interest in activities that you previously enjoyed are all symptoms pointing to depression. You may lose interest in your diabetes management activities when you are depressed. It is important to talk to your health care team about these feelings and changes in your life. Your physician may be able to recommend counselling or temporarily prescribe a medication that can help you enjoy life again.

*I*s there a list of tests and other things I am supposed to be doing to stay healthy?

Diabetes Checklist

Care Activities	Frequency	Date
Diabetes Control	Review BG log quarterly HbA$_{1c}$ goal _____	
Ophthalmology	Annual dilated exam Glaucoma, cataract check	
Renal	Proteinuria/microalbuminuria screen BUN/creatinine annual	
Neuropathy/Feet	Feet and legs quarterly Podiatry referral as needed	
Cardiovascular Exam	BP quarterly Lipids: annual screen fasting Get a baseline ECG	
Hypoglycemia/ Hyperglycemia	Review management plan Glucagon on hand?	
Vaccinations	Flu: annual Pneumovax	
Diabetes Education	Initial & annual review	
Other:	Hospitalizations: Dates? Reasons?	

▼

TIP:

Yes. The ADA publishes "Standards of Medical Care for Patients with Diabetes Mellitus" to provide guidelines for health professionals to manage diabetes and prevent complications. We use a chart based on those standards to help our patients keep track of all that needs to be done. Some tests come every 3 months and some yearly. For instance, you should have your eyes checked by an ophthalmologist and your urine checked for microalbuminuria (small amounts of protein) yearly. With these two tests, we can detect eye and kidney problems early and start treatment. You may want to keep your own flow chart to be sure to get the tests done at the right time and to be able to share these results with your health care team. Talk with them about which tests you need and when to have each one done.

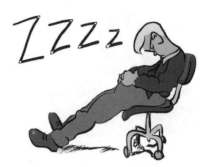

*W*hy do I sleep all the time and yet never feel rested?

▼
TIP:

There are a number of reasons for someone to feel tired and want to sleep all the time. If your blood sugar is too high, it may make you very sleepy and make you lack energy. You may get very sleepy after eating a meal, a feeling that might be caused by an increase in your blood sugar. Your tiredness may be a side effect from your medications. Medicines associated with making you feel tired are some ulcer medications, antihistamines, blood pressure medications, treatments for stomach emptying problems (gastroparesis), and most antidepressants. Ask your pharmacist or physician whether any of your medications could be causing your tiredness. You may have a thyroid problem that shows up as tiredness. Finally, you may be depressed and not realize it. Many people with depression sleep excessive numbers of hours and yet never feel rested. Other symptoms of depression include loss of appetite, disinterest in activities that you once enjoyed, and frequent crying spells. Talk to your health care team about these symptoms. There are simple ways to identify depression and good treatments available.

Why does a doctor have to sign my driver's license application?*

▼
TIP:

This is so doctors can identify people who should not be driving for medical reasons. People with diabetes may endanger themselves and others if their eyesight is badly impaired because of diabetic eye disease. They may also suffer from frequent and severe low blood sugars that may interfere with their ability to operate an automobile. This risk is low, however, with only one out of every 10,000 automobile accidents being attributable to low blood sugar (a rate that is 1,000 times less than the risk of an alcohol-related accident). The best general approach to renewing your driver's license is to establish a relationship with your health care team so that they know how well you manage your diabetes. In most cases, your physician will review your files and sign the form, agreeing that your license should be renewed. If there is a question about your eyesight, you may be sent to an eye doctor for evaluation. If your doctor feels that your blood sugar control is too erratic for you to operate an automobile safely, you may need to learn more about managing your diabetes responsibly. The potential loss of your driver's license may become the motivator you need to take charge of your diabetes!

*This is not required in all states.

Why does it hurt when my husband and I have sex?

▼
TIP:

Although men with diabetes more commonly have sexual problems, women may also experience sexual difficulties caused by the disease. These problems may include a decrease in sexual desire, vaginal dryness and pain with intercourse, or inability to achieve orgasm. Complaints such as these are not unique to people with diabetes but tend to occur more often in women with diabetes, especially those who are past menopause. Loss of sexual desire may be a symptom of depression. It frequently responds to medication or a few visits with a therapist. Some women have an increase in sexual desire after treatment with low-dose testosterone (a hormone). Your pain during intercourse, however, most likely is caused by vaginal dryness and the fact that your sex organs don't always adequately prepare for the sex act. If you are entering or past menopause, this problem may improve with estrogen replacement therapy or an estrogen cream that you put into the vagina. The use of sexual lubricants may also greatly improve your enjoyment of sex. Talking about your concern with your health care team may help you resume a fulfilling and mutually satisfying sex life with your husband.

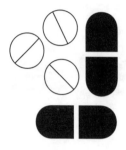

*I*s there any birth control method that
is preferred because I have diabetes?

▼
TIP:

You and your health care team need to decide which birth
control method will work best for you. You should use
some kind of birth control if you are sexually active and don't
want to get pregnant. Birth control pills contain very low levels
of estrogen (a hormone), and you can use them. You may need
more insulin, because the hormones in the birth control pills
might make you a bit more insulin resistant. A combination
pill with norgestinate and a synthetic estrogen is the best one
for women with diabetes. Foam, condoms, or a diaphragm
work well as long as you use them every time. Condoms also
provide the extra benefit of protection from sexually transmit-
ted diseases, such as AIDS. If you want a birth control method
that requires little effort, there are hormone "implants" and
injections. These provide birth control over a longer period of
time, but they do affect your diabetes control. Another option
for some women is the IUD (intrauterine device), which is a
small plastic device placed inside the uterus that prevents
implantation of fertilized eggs. Because they can increase your
chances of developing an infection, IUDs are not recommended
for women with diabetes.

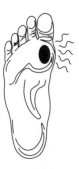

*I*f my feet don't hurt, should I still check
them every day?

▼
TIP:

Yes! You should examine your feet at the end of each day
to be certain that there are no sores, cuts, or areas where
your shoe is rubbing against your foot. People with diabetes
may lose pain sensation in their feet, so they may develop
ulcers and open sores and not notice it because they can't feel
the pain. Without medical attention, sores may continue to be
irritated and not heal properly. Although your health care team
should examine your feet at each visit, you need to be on the
lookout for any small areas of redness or bleeding. It is essential
that your shoes be comfortable and fit well. Special shoes can
be made for you if your feet are difficult to fit. Always wear
socks or stockings to provide padding between your feet and
your shoes. The longer a patient has diabetes, the more common foot problems are. Preventing foot sores is much easier
than trying to heal them.

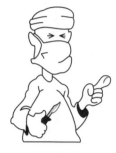

My doctor says that I should have my gallbladder removed, but isn't there a high risk of surgical complications because of my diabetes?

▼
TIP:

Patients with diabetes are at a higher risk of complications during and after a surgical procedure, but many such patients undergo successful surgery every day. Assuming that your surgery is necessary, then it is most important that your surgeon and your diabetes doctor work together before the surgery is performed to prevent problems. You should have a thorough medical checkup of your heart and kidneys, and you should make sure that your blood sugar control is good over the weeks prior to surgery. You should also be sure that you have had plenty of fluids to drink before reporting to the hospital. During the surgery, your doctors may control your blood sugar with intravenous insulin and glucose. Your diabetes doctor may even wish to be present during the surgery. After surgery, tight blood sugar control helps you reduce the risk of post-operative infections. By taking these precautions, you will have the best chances for a successful operation.

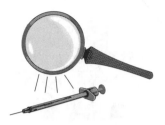

*H*ow can I accurately measure
1/2-unit doses of insulin for my
2-year-old son who has diabetes?

▼
TIP:

It is helpful to use low-dose (50 unit) or very-low-dose (30 unit) syringes when measuring small amounts of insulin because these syringes are narrower and have an expanded scale on the barrel. Syringe attachments that magnify and make it easier to read the scale are also available in many pharmacies. In addition, insulin manufacturers will provide diluting fluid if necessary for more accurate measurement.

Many children are extremely sensitive to insulin, and it is not unusual for doctors to prescribe 1/2-unit doses of insulin for such patients. One recent study determined how accurately the parents (caretakers) of young children with diabetes were able to prepare very small doses of insulin. The results of this study suggest that people do not measure insulin very accurately in 1/2-unit doses. Interestingly, the study also found that people tend to overestimate the dose and deliver more insulin than they are supposed to. The good news is that each person tends to overestimate by the same amount nearly every time. So to keep measurements consistent, small children with diabetes may need to have only one caretaker who prepares their insulin injections.

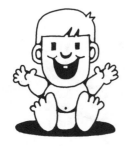

What are the risks to my baby during my pregnancy?

TIP:

Pregnancy in diabetes carries risks for both you and your baby. Babies born of diabetic mothers have higher rates of birth defects and stillbirth. They can also be abnormally large, which complicates the delivery. You can avoid many of these problems by achieving near-normal blood sugar control before and during pregnancy. For example, infants born of diabetic mothers have about a 10% chance of being born with a birth defect, compared with only 2% of babies born to nondiabetic mothers. These birth defects typically involve the spinal cord, the kidneys, and the heart. This risk of birth defects can be greatly reduced, however, by achieving normal blood sugar control before pregnancy even occurs. In fact, blood sugar control is most important during the first 12 weeks of pregnancy because this is the time when all of the infant's major organs are formed. To be safe, you should plan on achieving a glycated hemoglobin (HbA_{1c}) level within 1% of normal before you start trying to get pregnant. If successful, you will give your baby the best chance for a healthy start in life, and you will also decrease the chances of delivering a very large baby. This will improve your chances of staying healthy, too.

If I am hospitalized, what should I expect regarding my diabetes care?

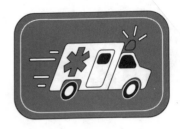

▼
TIP:

Your blood sugar control may worsen in the hospital because of varying content and timing of meals, inactivity, the stress of being in the hospital, and changes in your insulin dose. The physician might not know your diabetes as well as you do. Stay involved in your diabetes care (assuming that you feel well enough). Measure your blood sugar yourself and keep a record by your bedside so that you can discuss your blood sugar levels with your doctor. Your blood sugar should be measured at least four times a day. Your doctor should establish a target range for you, usually less than 200 mg/dl. Expect your insulin or oral diabetes medication at a reasonable time (always before meals). If you feel that you are not getting enough food, ask for more and tell your doctor. If you are unable to eat, expect your diabetes to be controlled by insulin given in your IV. This will require frequent monitoring of your blood sugar to ensure that it does not go too low or too high. You should also expect the doctor to check your urine ketones more frequently in the hospital than you do at home, because fasting and stress can both lead to ketoacidosis. Taking an active role in your own diabetes care in the hospital will increase your chances of staying healthy.

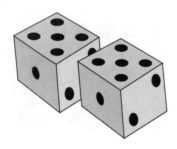

If I have "impaired glucose tolerance," what are my chances of getting diabetes later in life?

▼
TIP:

Impaired glucose tolerance (IGT) is a dangerous pre-diabetic condition. Reversing it with diet and exercise may prevent you from getting diabetes. Impaired glucose tolerance is a gray area between having normal blood sugar and having diabetes. If you have IGT, your pre-breakfast blood sugar values are slightly elevated, usually above 110 mg/dl. This level is not high enough to qualify for a diagnosis of diabetes, which is above 126 mg/dl. Although you don't have diabetes, 5% of people with IGT do develop diabetes every year. This means that if you have had IGT for 5 years, your chances for getting diabetes increase to about 25%. People with IGT are usually overweight, don't get much exercise, and often have relatives who have type 2 diabetes. Most doctors believe that if people with IGT improve their health by losing weight and getting more exercise, their chance of developing diabetes will be much lower. Also, eating a low-fat and high-fiber diet may help. You should get your blood sugar level checked at least once a year, and if it is high, go to work on getting it into the normal range and keeping it there.

Chapter 8
NEW TIPS

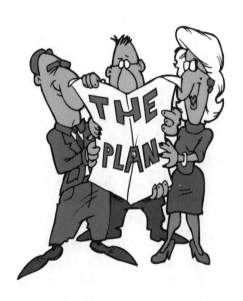

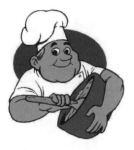

Should I use the new artificial sweetener Splenda instead of the other available sweeteners?

▼
TIP:

Splenda (sucralose) is a new, noncaloric sweetener recently approved by the FDA. It has several advantages over previously approved artificial sweeteners. First, to date it has shown no toxicity in humans, although long-term studies in humans are not yet available. Second, it is noncaloric and approximately five times sweeter than table sugar. Third, it is much more stable than either Nutrasweet or Equal when used in cooking and baking. Fourth, Splenda tastes like sugar and has no unpleasant aftertaste. For these reasons, Splenda will undoubtedly become very popular as an artificial sweetener. However, whether or not you should use it will depend on its price in the supermarket and on concern that long-term studies in humans proving its safety are not yet available. However, to date, animals given high doses of Splenda have shown no adverse effects.

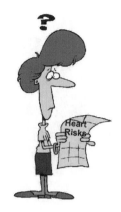

Should I take an aspirin daily if I have diabetes?

▼
TIP:

Probably. Diabetes increases your risk of dying from complications of heart and cardiovascular disease, so this is a reasonable question to ask. In November 1997, the ADA concluded that low-dose aspirin therapy should be prescribed not only in patients with diabetes who have had heart attacks, but also in patients with diabetes who are at a high risk for future heart and artery disease. This includes both men and women. The reason that people with diabetes may be at greater risk is that their platelets (parts of cells circulating around in the blood that clump and prevent bleeding) may clump more spontaneously than in people who do not have diabetes. Aspirin prevents this clumping and therefore may prevent heart attacks. Taking aspirin, however, is not without risk. It can cause stomach and intestinal bleeding. That's why people with bleeding ulcers shouldn't take aspirin. However, this risk is greatly reduced if you take enteric-coated aspirin of 81–325 mg a day. In fact, the lower dose (81 mg) of enteric-coated aspirin has been shown to be just as effective as any higher doses in preventing platelets from clumping. You should discuss the use of aspirin with your physician to make sure that it's safe for you.

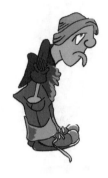

How can my adolescent son or daughter learn to be happy in spite of having diabetes?

▼
TIP:

S tudies have shown that adolescents with diabetes have lower "quality of life" scores and are more prone to depression than teenagers who don't have diabetes. One recent study, however, suggests that a brief period of training in "coping skills" can improve both an adolescent's quality of life score and his or her diabetes control. Such training involves unlearning bad coping skills (such as eating too much or denying the problem) that everyone uses to deal with stressful circumstances. The adolescent then learns new skills that give him or her healthier, more productive ways to react to stress. In the study, these skills were taught by trained professionals in four to eight 90-minute sessions over 1 month. Adolescents who received the coping skills training showed improvement in scores that measured their confidence in managing diabetes, tendency to depression, and overall quality of life. Teenagers who received training in coping skills also had lower blood sugar levels than those who did not. Ask your son or daughter's diabetes care provider how your child can receive coping skills training.

*W̶hat will help heal the ulcers
on my feet?*

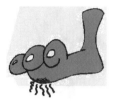

▼
TIP:

Healing requires good foot care from your health provider, including antibiotics and removal of the dead tissue. You do your part by not walking on the foot, keeping it clean and dry, and following your health care team's guidance.

A new medication called Regranex gel (becaplermin) has recently been approved by the FDA for use on foot ulcers that have adequate blood vessels going to them. This medication enhances new blood vessel formation and healing of your ulcer. It is made by recombinant gene technology and not directly from blood products and therefore is probably safer than if it were made directly from blood.

If you use this medication, there are several steps you should consider. First, before applying the gel, your ulcer must be clean and all nonliving tissue must be removed by your physician or podiatrist. Healing may begin within 2 weeks and be completed in 10 weeks. Studies in patients with diabetes show that using Regranex is better than using good ulcer care alone. Regranex healed approximately 50% of the ulcers compared to 30–40% healed with standard care alone. Unfortunately, this medication is very expensive. Hopefully, the price will drop in the future. This medication may give you the extra assistance you need, but your foot still requires careful care and close follow-up with your physician.

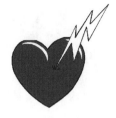

How high is my risk for heart attack with type 2 diabetes?

TIP:

Higher than you might think! In people who don't have diabetes, one of the strongest predictors for the development of a heart attack is a previous heart attack. A recent study has shown that people with type 2 diabetes who have not had a heart attack still have as high a risk for a future heart attack as a person without diabetes who has already had a heart attack. In other words, your risk for a future heart attack is as high as the risk for a person without diabetes who has known heart disease. This finding suggests that risk factors for heart disease, such as smoking, high blood pressure, and high blood cholesterol levels, should be treated very aggressively in people with diabetes. Some experts even feel that people with type 2 diabetes should be treated with medication as if they already have heart disease. So if your diabetes care team suggests specific treatment to lower your risk of heart attack, you should strongly consider giving it a try.

*I*s insulin resistance important to my diabetes? What can I do about it?

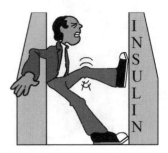

▼
TIP:

Yes, insulin resistance makes diabetes worse. We don't know why people with diabetes have insulin resistance. Physicians recommend several ways to reduce insulin resistance to make your own insulin more effective and better able to control your blood sugar. The nondrug ways to reduce insulin resistance are a low-calorie diet, weight loss, and regular and vigorous exercise. In other words, a healthy lifestyle can help you reduce insulin resistance. Recently, two medications have been approved by the FDA for type 2 diabetes. These two drugs also reduce insulin resistance and therefore improve diabetes control. Metformin (Glucophage) acts on your liver and, to a lesser extent, on your muscles to reduce insulin resistance. Troglitazone (Rezulin) has been shown to act in the liver, muscles, and fat tissue to reduce insulin resistance. These two medications are widely used in the management of type 2 diabetes and have been shown to be very effective. If you have type 2 diabetes, discuss with your health provider which approaches are best for you to reduce the insulin resistance in your body.

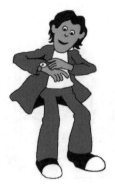

When should I take my lispro insulin injection if my blood sugar is high before a meal?

▼
TIP:

Lispro (Humalog) is a rapid-acting insulin, so it is recommended that you take it 0–15 minutes before eating a meal. However, this advice may not apply if you have high blood sugars. You may need to inject and wait for your blood sugar to come down before eating. This will ensure lower blood sugars after eating. A recent study examined the effect of varying the timing of the lispro insulin injection before breakfast in people who had blood sugars of 180 mg/dl. This study showed that for 5 hours after breakfast, blood sugars remained lower when the lispro insulin was injected 15 or 30 minutes before eating compared with an injection right at mealtime. Lispro insulin is a significant advance in insulin therapy and allows you to correct high blood sugars much more rapidly than if you use regular insulin. However, it is good to be aware of the need for proper timing of the lispro insulin injection if you have high blood sugars before mealtime.

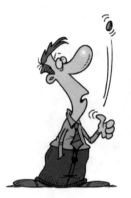

Can diabetes complications be predicted?

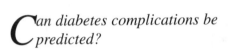

▼
TIP:

Sometimes. We know that certain factors, such as having consistently high blood sugar levels, predict the development of more diabetic complications, but we cannot predict who will get which complications. Still, research studies on complications can be useful and informative. For example, one recent study attempted to determine the most important predictors for eye disease, kidney disease, and amputation among 2,774 patients with diabetes. This study showed that older individuals and people who had less education were more likely to suffer complications. But other factors were also important. In people with type 1 diabetes, the combination of high blood pressure and smoking was the most powerful predictor of diabetic complications. For people with type 2 diabetes, failure to seek regular diabetes care was the most powerful predictor of diabetic complications. Although we can never be absolutely certain that you will not develop diabetic complications, we do know that you can minimize your risk by carefully controlling your blood sugar, controlling your blood pressure, quitting smoking, and working with your diabetes care team to be as healthy as you can be.

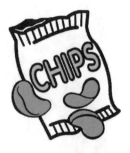

*W*hat are "fat replacers"?

▼
TIP:

Fat replacers are ingredients that manufacturers put in food to play the role of some of the fat in that food. These "replacers" can be made of carbohydrate, protein, or fat. The reason that fat replacers may be advantageous to your diet is the simple fact that fat contains 9 calories per gram of food, a very high energy content for a small amount of food. (Carbohydrate and protein have only 4 calories per gram.) On the other hand, many fat replacers, particularly if they are carbohydate- or protein-based, contain only 5 calories per gram of food. So, if you eat the same weight of food, you actually get half as many calories and might therefore lose weight. The problem is that many people assume that fat-free foods are so much lower in calories that they can eat larger servings of them. This is not the case; fat free does not mean calorie free. Also, watch for fat replacers that are made of carbohydrate because they will have an effect on your blood sugar level.

How should I manage my diabetes during a prolonged fast such as for Ramadan?

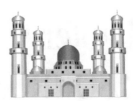

▼
TIP:

Ramadan is a month-long fast observed by the Muslim religion. Whether or not you should participate is a subject of controversy among diabetes care providers, but we recognize that many patients will participate. First of all, recognize that food intake is not totally prohibited during Ramadan. It is only prohibited during daylight hours. Many patients with type 2 diabetes may be able to develop a schedule to meet these requirements, although dosages of certain diabetes medications may have to be decreased or stopped during this period. Prolonged fasting represents a more difficult problem for people with type 1 diabetes. Insulin doses will probably have to be greatly reduced to avoid low blood sugar, and frequent blood sugar monitoring is essential. Ketones are produced with fasting and insulin deficiency, so check urine ketones once or twice a day to avoid developing dangerous ketoacidosis. Ask your doctor what to do if ketones appear in your urine, but you don't have high blood sugar. Finally, develop a plan for treating hypoglycemia while you are fasting. The Muslim religion exempts people who are ill from strict fasting, so it may be reasonable to decide to eat something if your blood sugar drops below some predetermined threshold, such as 60 mg/dl.

Chapter 9
RESOURCES

American Association of Diabetes Educators . . . . . .(800) 338-3633
444 N. Michigan Ave.   (312) 644-2233
Suite 1240
Chicago, IL 60611-3901

American Diabetes Association . . . .(800) 806-7801
Patient Information   (800) 342-2383
1660 Duke St.   (703) 549-1500
Alexandria, VA 22314

The American Dietetic Association . . . .(800) 366-1655
216 West Jackson Blvd.
Suite 800
Chicago, IL 60606-6995

International Diabetic Athletes Association . . . .(602) 230-8155
6829 North 12th St.
Suite 205
Phoenix, AZ 85014

National Diabetes Information Clearinghouse . . . . .(301) 468-2162
Box NDIC
9000 Rockville Pk.
Bethesda, MD 20892

INDEX

sodium intake, lowering, 58
weight reduction programs, 61
Dipyridamole stress test, 84
Disclosure, of diabetes, 2
Dizziness, 82
Doctor visits
checklist for, 98
frequency of, 7, 68, 89, 98
for heart disease screening, 84
preparation for, 6
Docusate, 95
Driving
blood glucose testing before, 43
commercial vehicles, insulin use
and, 25
license renewal, 100

E
Erectile dysfunction, 19
Erections, maintaining, 83
Erythromycin, 24
Estrogen, 101
Exercise
arthritis and, 33
athletic shoes, 80
benefits, 33
blood glucose testing before, 43
to decrease blood pressure, 96
and IGT, reversing, 108
laser therapy and, 77
stopping medication and, 45
Eye problems, 68
assessments, 7
blindness, 13, 68, 72
glaucoma, 72
infections, 72
pregnancy and, 69
temporary loss of vision, 82

F
Fainting spells, 82
Family members, reading this book,
8
Fasting, 62, 119
Fat, dietary, 90
Fat replacers, 118

Fatigue, 36, 97, 99
Fiber, dietary, 49, 95
diabetic gastroparesis and, 71
Finger joints, stiffness in, 74
Fingernails, fungal infections of, 20
Finger sticks, reducing pain of, 35
Fish oil, 42
Floaters, 68
Florinef, 82
Folate, 53
Folic acid, 53
Food and Drug Administration, 15,
19, 21, 52, 59, 110, 115
Food guide pyramid, 60
Food labeling, 59
Foot care, 22, 85–86, 113
athlete's foot, 20
daily examination, 103
painful neuropathy, 74
shoes, 80, 103
Frank, Johann Peter, 14
Fructose, 50
Fungal infections, 20, 23

G
Ginseng, 51–52
Glaucoma, 72
Glipizide, 46
Glucophage, 21
Glucose control. *See* Blood glucose
levels
Glucose sensors, 4
Glucose testing. *See* Blood glucose
testing
Glyburide, 46
Glycated hemoglobin (HbA$_{1c}$), 67
level for pregnancy, 106
Gustatory sweating, 78

H
Hands, stiffness in, 75
Health care team, 11. *See also* Doctor
visits
Health foods, 49–55
Health insurance

pancreas transplants and, 39
preexisting condition exclusion, 18
Health management. *See also* Doctor
  visits
  coworkers and, 2
  test guidelines, 98
Heart disease
  aspirin and, 111
  cholesterol and, 87
  fat intake and, 90
  homocysteine and, 53
  hot tubs and, 88
  risk of, 81, 91, 114
  saunas and, 88
  syndrome X, 91
  testing for, 84
  waist/hip ratio and, 65
Hemoglobin, glycated, 67, 106
Hepatitis, 35
Herbal remedies, 52
Heredity, as cause of diabetes, 3, 16
High blood glucose. *See also* Blood
  glucose levels
  damage from, 44
Historical background, diabetes, 10,
  14
Homocysteine, 53
Hospitalization
  blood glucose control and, 107
  surgery, 104
Hot tubs, 88

I
Impaired glucose tolerance (IGT),
  108
Incontinence, 89
Infections
  eye, 72
  foot, 22, 86, 113
  from IUDs, 102
  postoperative, 104
  skin, 23
Infectiousness, of diabetes, 3
Insoluble fiber, 49
Insulin
  allergic reaction to, 42

birth control pills and, 102
blood glucose testing and, 43
discovery of, 10
driving commercial vehicles and, 25
lispro, 116
low dosages for children, 105
resistance, 115
weight gain and, 46
Insulin-dependent diabetes. *See* type 1
  diabetes
Insulin pumps, 4, 37
Internet, diabetes information on, 27
IUD (intrauterine device), 102

K
Kaopectate, 24
Ketoacidosis, 26, 62, 107
Ketones, 26, 62, 107, 119
Kidneys
  assessments of, 7
  blood pressure medication and, 93
  failure of, 13
  problems during pregnancy, 69, 73
  protein and, 76
  transplants of, 39

L
Langerhans, Paul, 10
Laser therapy, 68
  exercise following, 77
Leg cramps, 74
Lispro insulin, 116
Lomotil, 24
Loperamide, 24
Losartan, 93
Low blood glucose, 36. *See also*
  Blood glucose levels

M
Macular edema, 68
Magnesium supplements, 54
Meal planning. *See also* Diet
  adherence to, 63
  frequency of meals, 64
Medical costs, 18
  insulin pumps, 37

Smoking, 81, 117
Sodium, lowering intake of, 58, 96
Soluble fiber, 49
Spilling protein, 76
Splenda, 110
Standards of Medical Care for
  Patients with Diabetes Mellitus, 98
Stiffness, in hands, 75
Stomach problems, 71
Stress tests, 84
Strokes, homocysteine and, 53
Summer camps, 30
Supervisors, diabetes disclosure and,
  2
Supplements, dietary, 48
  folic acid (folate), 53
  ginseng, 51–52
  herbal remedies, 52
  magnesium, 54
  melatonin, 55
  vanadium, 52
Support groups, 11
Surgery, 104, 107. *See also*
  Transplants
Sweating, gustatory, 78
Syndrome X, 91
Syringes, low-dose, 105

T
Teenagers, diabetes care and, 30
Testosterone, 83, 101
Tetracycline, 24
Thyroid problems, 5
  constipation and, 95
Tiredness, 36, 97, 99
TOPS (Take Off Pounds Sensibly),
  61
Transplants
  of insulin-producing cells, 4
  of pancreas, 39
Triglyceride levels, 42, 90, 91
Type 1 diabetes
  causes of, 3, 16
  ketoacidosis, 62
  occurrence, 17
  prevention of, 16

Type 2 diabetes
  causes of, 3, 16
  dietary fiber and, 49
  ginseng and, 51–52
  heart attack risk and, 114
  occurrence, 17
  oral medications, 21
  prevention of, 16, 108
  stopping medication, 45

U
Urine leakage, 89
Urine testing, 26

V
Vaginal dryness, 101
Vanadium, 52
Viagra, 19
Viral conjunctivitis, 72
Vision. *See* Eye problems
Vitamin supplements. *See*
  Supplements, dietary

W
Waist/hip ratio, 65
Weight control, 46, 115, 118
  age and, 94
  diet/weight reduction programs, 61
  and IGT, reversing, 108
  obesity, 91
  syndrome X, 90
  waist/hip ratio, 65
Weight Watchers, 61
White classification, 69
Wine, 34
World Wide Web, diabetes
  information on, 27

Y
Yawning, 36
Yeast infections, 23
Yohimbine, 83

More Books from the
American Diabetes Association

New!
101 Medication Tips for People with Diabetes
Mary Anne Koda-Kimble, PharmD, CDE
Betsy A. Carlisle, PharmD
Lisa Kroon, PharmD

1. What is the difference between regular and lispro insulin?
2. What are the main side effects of the drugs used to treat type 2 diabetes?
3. Will my diabetes medications interact with other drugs I'm taking?
4. My doctor prescribed an "ACE inhibitor." What is this drug? What will it do?

Treating diabetes can get complicated, especially when you consider the bewildering number of medications that must be carefully integrated with diet and exercise. Here you'll find answers to 101 of the most commonly asked questions about diabetes and medication. An indispensable reference for anyone with type 1, type 2, or gestational diabetes.

One Low Price: $14.95
Order #4833-01

New!
101 Nutrition Tips for People with Diabetes
Patti B. Geil, MS, RD, FADA, CDE
Lea Ann Holzmeister, RD, CDE

1. Which type of fiber helps my blood sugar?
2. What do I do if my toddler refuses to eat her meal?
3. If a food is sugar-free, can I eat all I want?

In this latest addition to the best-selling 101 Tips series, co-authors Patti Geil and Lea Ann Holzmeister—experts on nutrition and diabetes—use their professional experience with hundreds of patients over the years to answer the most commonly asked questions about diabetes and nutrition. You'll discover handy tips on meal planning, general nutrition, managing medication and meals, shopping and cooking, weight loss, and more.

One Low Price: $14.95
Order #4828-01

Newly Revised!
101 Tips for Staying Healthy with Diabetes (& Avoiding Complications),
2nd Edition
David S. Schade, MD
and The University of New Mexico Diabetes Care Team

1. Is testing your urine for glucose and ketones an accurate way to measure blood sugar?
2. What's the best way to reduce the pain of frequent finger sticks?
3. Will an insulin pump help you prevent complications?

These are just a few of the more than 110 tips you'll discover in this newly revised second edition of an ADA bestseller. Dozens of other tips—many of them just added—will help you reduce the risk of complications and ensure a healthy life.

One Low Price: $14.95
Order #4810-01

New!
The Diabetes Problem Solver
Nancy Touchette, PhD

Quick: You think you may have diabetic ketoacidosis, a life-threatening condition. What are the symptoms? What should you do first? What are the treatments? How could it have been prevented? *The Diabetes Problem Solver* is the first reference guide that helps you identify and prevent the most common diabetes-related problems you encounter from day-to-day. From hypoglycemia, nerve pain, and foot ulcers to eye disease, depression, and eating disorders, virtually every possible problem is covered. And the solutions are at your fingertips. *The Problem Solver* addresses each problem by answering five crucial questions:

1. What's the problem?
2. Do I have the symptoms?
3. What should I do?
4. What's the best treatment?

You'll find extensive, easy-to-read coverage of just about every diabetes problem you can imagine, and comprehensive flowcharts at the front of the book lead you from symptoms to possible solutions quickly.

One Low Price: $19.95
Order #4825-01

New!
Diabetes Meal Planning on $7 a Day—or Less
Patti B. Geil, MS, RD, FADA, CDE
Tami A. Ross, RD, CDE

You can save money—lots of it—without sacrificing what's most important to you: a healthy variety of great-tasting meals. Learn how to save money by planning meals more carefully, use shopping tips to save money at the grocery store, eat at your favorite restaurants economically, and much more. Each of the 100 quick and easy recipes includes cost-per-serving and complete nutrition information to help you create a more cost-conscious, healthy meal plan.

One Low Price: $12.95
Order #4711-01

New!
Meditations on Diabetes
Catherine Feste

Modern medicine has come full circle to realize again what ancient healers knew: that illness affects both the body and the soul. Cathy Feste has lived with diabetes for 40 years, so she knows the physical, emotional, and spiritual challenges that come with diabetes. With every turn of the page you'll discover reassuring advice and insight in daily meditations from the author's journals with a little help from her friends, such as Ralph Waldo Emerson, Eleanor Roosevelt, Helen Keller, and many others.

One Low Price: $13.95
Order #4820-01

When Diabetes Hits Home
Wendy Satin Rapaport, LCSW, PsyD

A reassuring exploration of the full spectrum of emotional issues you and your family may struggle with throughout your lives. You'll learn how to cope with the initial period of anger and anxiety at diagnosis, develop your spiritual self and discover the meaning of living with a chronic disease, address the changes all families go through and learn how to cope with them emotionally, and much more.

One Low Price: $19.95
Order #4818-01

The Uncomplicated Guide to Diabetes Complications
Edited by Marvin E. Levin, MD
and Michael A. Pfeifer, MD

Thorough, comprehensive chapters cover everything you need to know about preventing and treating diabetes complications—in simple language that anyone can understand. All major complications and special concerns are covered, including kidney disease, heart disease, obesity, eye disease and blindness, impotence and sexual disorders, hypertension and stroke, neuropathy and vascular disease, and more.

One Low Price: $18.95
Order #4814-01

Women & Diabetes
Laurinda M. Poirier, RN, MPH, CDE
Katherine M. Coburn, MPH

A woman's life is complex enough with all the roles that she plays during her lifetime. Diabetes compounds the complexity and challenges a woman mentally, physically, and spiritually. This book, written by two health professionals—one of whom has diabetes—offers special thoughts to help you move through life with confidence.

Nonmember: $14.95
Member: $13.95
Order #4907-01

Caring for the Diabetic Soul
Simple solutions for coping with the psychological challenges of diabetes.

Nonmember: $9.95
Member: $8.95
Order #4815-01

Winning with Diabetes
Inspiring true stories of people who live life to the fullest, despite having diabetes.

One Low Price: $12.95
Order #4824-01

Dear Diabetes Advisor
Michael A. Pfeifer, MD, CDE

Solid, no-nonsense answers to commonsense questions about diabetes.

Nonmember: $9.95
Member: $8.95
Order #4813-01

Best-seller!
American Diabetes Association Complete Guide to Diabetes
Everything you want to know about diabetes, a guide packed with ideas, tips, and techniques for dealing with all types of diabetes.

Nonmember: $19.95
Member: $15.95
Order #4809-01

Revised Best-seller!
Type 2 Diabetes: Your Healthy Living Guide, 2nd Edition
A thorough guide to staying healthy with type 2 diabetes.

Nonmember: $16.95
Member: $14.95
Order #4804-01

New!
The Great Chicken Cookbook for People with Diabetes
Beryl M. Marton

Now you can have chicken any way you want it—and healthy too! More than 150 great-tasting, low-fat chicken recipes in all, including baked chicken, braised chicken, chicken casseroles, grilled chicken, rolled and stuffed chicken, chicken soups, chicken stir-fry, chicken with pasta, and many more.

One Low Price: $16.95
Order #4627-01

New!

The New Soul Food Cookbook for People with Diabetes
Fabiola Demps Gaines, RD, LD
Roneice Weaver, RD, LD

Dig into sensational low-fat recipes from the first African-American cookbook
for people with diabetes. More than 150 recipes in all, including shrimp
jambalaya, fried okra, orange sweet potatoes, corn muffins, apple crisp, and
many more.

One Low Price: $14.95
Order #4623-01

New!

The Diabetes Snack Munch Nibble Nosh Book
Ruth Glick

Choose from 150 low-sodium, low-fat snacks and mini-meals, such as pizza
puffs, mustard pretzels, apple-cranberry turnovers, bread puzzle, cinnamon
biscuits and pecan buns, alphabet letters, banana pops, and many others.
Special features include recipes for one or two and snack ideas for hard-to-
please kids. Nutrient analyses, preparation times, and exchanges are included
with every recipe.

One Low Price: $14.95
Order Code: #4622-01

The ADA Guide to Healthy Restaurant Eating
Hope S. Warshaw, MMSc, RD, CDE

Finally! One book with all the facts you need to eat out intelligently—whether
you're enjoying burgers, pizza, bagels, pasta, or burritos at your favorite
restaurant. Special features include more than 2,500 menu items from more
than 50 major restaurant chains, complete nutrition information for every
menu item, restaurant pitfalls and strategies for defensive restaurant dining,
and much more.

One Low Price: $13.95
Order #4819-01

About the American Diabetes Association

The American Diabetes Association is the nation's leading voluntary health organization supporting diabetes research, information, and advocacy. Founded in 1940, the Association provides services to communities across the country. Its mission is to prevent and cure diabetes and to improve the lives of all people affected by diabetes.

For more than 50 years, the American Diabetes Association has been the leading publisher of comprehensive diabetes information for people with diabetes and the health care professionals who treat them. Its huge library of practical and authoritative books for people with diabetes covers every aspect of self care—cooking and nutrition, fitness, weight control, medications, complications, emotional issues, and general self care. The Association also publishes books and medical treatment guides for physicians and other health care professionals.

Membership in the Association is available to health care professionals and people with diabetes and includes subscriptions to one or more of the Association's periodicals. People with diabetes receive *Diabetes Forecast*, the nation's leading health and wellness magazine for people with diabetes. Health care professionals receive one or more of the Association's five scientific and medical journals.

For more information, please call toll-free:

Questions about diabetes:	1-800-DIABETES
Membership, people with diabetes:	1-800-806-7801
Membership, health professionals:	1-800-232-3472
Free catalog of ADA books:	1-800-232-6733
Visit us on the Web:	www.diabetes.org
Visit us at our Web bookstore:	merchant.diabetes.org